THE REVOLUTIONARY ANTI-AGING AND WEIGHT-LOSS PROGRAM FROM THE PRESTIGIOUS SOUTHWEST HEALTH INSTITUTE OF PHOENIX, ARIZONA

Safe, effective, medically sound, this total-body approach to looking and feeling younger offers amazing benefits—increased energy, prevention and improvement of health problems, and an active mental, physical, and sexual life for decades to come!

- Complete anti-aging diet
- No calorie counting
- Over fifty recipes created by leading chefs
- Menu plans
- Shopping tips
- Exercise and fitness guidelines
- Life-span extension program
- Vitamin and mineral supplements
- The ten commandments of anti-aging
- Exercises for mental alertness
- A secret anti-aging formula

"This is no fad diet book. It's grounded in medical research, in nutritional science, and in the author's experience treating patients."
—*Scottsdale Progress*

DR. ART MOLLEN is a nationally renowned health expert and founder of the Southwest Health Institute in Phoenix, Arizona. He is also a triathlete and a syndicated health columnist. He has published two previous bestsellers, *Run for Your Life* and *The Mollen Method*. He practices in Phoenix and Scottsdale, Arizona.

Dr. Mollen's Anti-Aging Diet

The Breakthrough Program for Easy Weight Loss and Longevity

DR. ART MOLLEN

with Judith Sachs

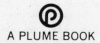

A PLUME BOOK

PLUME
Published by the Penguin Group
Penguin Books USA Inc., 375 Hudson Street, New York, New York 10014, U.S.A.
Penguin Books Ltd, 27 Wrights Lane, London W8 5TZ, England
Penguin Books Australia Ltd, Ringwood, Victoria, Australia
Penguin Books Canada Ltd, 10 Alcorn Avenue, Toronto, Ontario, Canada M4V 3B2
Penguin Books (N.Z.) Ltd, 182–190 Wairau Road, Auckland 10, New Zealand

Penguin Books Ltd, Registered Offices: Harmondsworth, Middlesex, England

Published by Plume, an imprint of New American Library,
a division of Penguin Books USA Inc. Previously published in a Dutton edition.

First Plume Printing, July, 1993
10 9 8 7 6 5 4 3 2 1   12/94

LIBRARY OF CONGRESS CATALOGING-IN-PUBLICATION DATA
Mollen, Art.
    Dr. Mollen's anti-aging diet : the breakthrough program for easy
weight loss and longevity / Art Mollen with Judith Sachs.
        p.   cm.
    Includes bibliographical references and index.
    ISBN 0-452-27055-3
    1. Reducing diets.   2. Low-protein diet.   3. Longevity.
I. Sachs, Judith.   II. Title.
RM222.2.M56   1993
613.2'5—dc20   92-45588
                                               CIP

Printed in the United States of America

Original hardcover design by Eve Kirch.

To my mom, not simply because she is my mother, but because she has taught me not to settle for less than the best at whatever I decided to accomplish.

A special note of gratitude and love to my wife, Molly, for helping me to make this book a more conscious contribution to society.

—A.M.

For my mother, Naomi, an actress of 78.
For my father, Milton, a physician of 81
—both of whom grow younger yearly.

—J.S.

ACKNOWLEDGMENTS

We thank Jean Merkel, the registered dietician who helped create the menus for the Anti-Aging Diet. She is a great contributor not only to this book but also to society.

We would also like to acknowledge the excellent recipe contributions of leading Phoenix chefs Vincent Guerithault of Vincent's on Camelback, Benito Mellino of Avanti's, Christopher Gross of Christopher's, and Chris Bianco of Bianco's.

We would like to express gratitude to every one of Dr. Mollen's patients, who helped us understand what the human body can achieve throughout the aging process.

We'd like to thank the brilliant researchers Dr. Linda Youngman at the University of California at Berkeley in the laboratory of Dr. Bruce Ames and Drs. Ronda Bell and Banoo Parpia at Cornell University in the laboratory of Dr. T. Colin Campbell. Their up-to-date studies on low-protein diets have been an invaluable aid in the work of the Southwest Health Clinic.

And finally, we would like to thank our editor, Michaela Hamilton, who guided the preparation of this book.

The doctor of the future will give no medicine, but will interest his patients in the care of the human frame, in diet, and in the cause and prevention of disease.

—Thomas Alva Edison

CONTENTS

Introduction

Wouldn't it be amazing if you were able to grow young instead of growing old? If you could feel completely energized each day now, in your thirties and forties and on into your nineties and hundreds? If you could live over a century in the absence of disease, growing stronger and healthier each day?

Well, it's not amazing. It's perfectly possible, and it won't require any superhuman effort on your part or bionic rebuilding in an expensive high-tech hospital. Whether you're 25 and want to sail through your days and nights with a new burst of energy or 45 and want to beat back those encroaching pounds and occasional twinges, you can make a positive difference—and I'm going to show you how.

A Diet that Really Works—Forever

My plan for you is a very simple one. All I want to do is give you the opportunity to grow younger and live longer—as a thinner, more energetic, happier person.

You don't have to feel exhausted and stressed-out after a day at

1

the office or racing after the kids. You can feel simply wonderful, refreshed and ready to go. And you don't have to dread the prospect of feeling sick and tired when you're 80 or even 100. Because my revolutionary Anti-Aging Diet is going to put zest into your present and incredible potential into your future.

You've probably been on countless diets over the years. You've lost weight and felt great. Then one day, the dull food and endless rules and regulations and feelings of deprivation and hunger got to you. You lost your motivation and figured, well, I can always start over again tomorrow. But tomorrow passed, and the next day, and you always had some excuse. Until the pounds and the depressed feeling returned, and you felt worse than ever.

This cyclical dieting defeat can't happen on my Anti-Aging Diet because it's not about quick fixes and temporary solutions. It is instead a continuum of good health, a way of life.

The Wave of the Future

We aren't very far into the '90s, but already the shape of the decade is becoming clear. As we approach the next century, we have to wipe the slate as clean as we can get it and establish new priorities. It's vital that we all become conscious of making choices that will lead to long-term gains. We're giving up frivolous fads for tested methods that will ensure a good today and a secure tomorrow for us all. The planet needs serious attention if we're going to keep it in good condition for another hundred years—and so do our life-styles and attitudes.

In the realm of health care, there's no time left for delay. It's urgent that we start taking better care of ourselves *now*, so that by the time we reach our centennials (and I'm going to see to it that we all do!) we won't have to give a thought to being sick and needing long-term care. In the twenty-first century, aging will take on a completely new image and be redefined as a goal we all strive for—not an event to be dreaded or feared.

But in order to be filled with vitality and power at 100, you have to start today, and you have to be open-minded, because my Anti-

Aging Diet is ground breaking in its thinking as well as its practical application. It is unlike any diet you've ever been on before. And it works.

There are currently more than 54,000 people over the age of 100 in America, and that number will be significantly greater by the year 2000. You may be one of them. But the Anti-Aging Diet is not just designed to add years to your life. It's going to start immediately to change your feelings about the way you approach eating, dieting, exercising and living. It's going to make every one of your hundred-plus years fulfilling, exciting and challenging.

Living to 120

Sometimes I get resistance from my patients about these goals. I remember when Nick first came to visit the Southwest Health Institute, the preventive health center I run in Phoenix, Arizona. He was 40, out of breath, overweight and his blood pressure was astronomically high. "I'm on the downhill slide, Doc, but if you can just get me to feel a little better and make it to 50, I'll be content."

I told him I probably wasn't the physician for him because I needed patients who didn't think of 40 as the end of the line but who had a real desire and motivation to live not just to 50 but to 100. And my goal for them was not only to make it there, but to arrive there joyously and easily. If he wanted to learn the essential truth of anti-aging and get there, too, he was going to have to work with me.

Six months later, thirty pounds lighter, with a now-normal blood pressure of 110/70, he told me my essential truth was ingenious and, yes, he'd like to stick around for six more decades—at the very least.

I don't know about you, but I don't intend to spend any of my money on hospital bills or long-term care facilities. I can't imagine myself retiring to go sit in the sun. I'm going to be much too busy for the next seventy years seeing patients, running several miles a day and enjoying life. How old am I now? Only 47.

You can live for 120 years, if you want to! Your body was brilliantly designed and engineered to withstand the stresses and strains of more than a century of use. Thanks to today's extraordinarily high level of medical achievement, we've been able to wipe out most of the deadly childhood diseases, control epidemics, and effect cures or remissions for many serious conditions that would have been fatal in past decades. So many patients who might have died at 50 or 60 from heart conditions or cancer are now cured. Unfortunately, medical science hasn't been able to fix everything. The rest is up to us. If we want to avoid debilitating old age, we have to consciously work to remain young and vital.

But what good is it to gain extra years if we can't live a rich, full existence every day? Aging doesn't have to mean getting old. It doesn't even have to mean retiring. Why should you give up what you've done just because you hit some magic number? Sixty-five is not the end of anything but the beginning of another twenty-five or thirty years of heightened productivity and pleasure. This pinnacle of life can be something you strive for now. You can start planning for the future, expand your goals, reach higher levels of energy and greater emotional maturity. You can become more than you've ever been in your life.

Reducing Protein to Live Longer

The reduction of protein in your diet is the most important element in weight loss and in slowing the aging process. On my Anti-Aging Diet, you will not only lose weight at a gradual and consistent rate and keep the weight off, you will also experience a rejuvenation of your body and mind. Since protein is taxing on the kidneys, liver, heart, and bones as you get older, you will actually stay younger by changing the balance of what you eat.

By eating only one portion of animal protein per day, you will effectively slow down your body's aging mechanism.

While you are on the weight-loss portion of this diet, you will consume 55 percent to 60 percent of your daily caloric intake in complex carbohydrates, 20 percent to 25 percent in fats, and about

20 percent in protein. As you progress to the anti-aging lifetime diet, your percentage of calories from protein will gradually decrease to between 10 percent and 12 percent of your daily calories. Most Americans consume about 40 percent of their daily calories in fats, and about the same in protein, leaving the sad remainder of only 20 percent to the most important foods—the complex carbohydrates, found in fruits, vegetables, legumes, and grains. We have all become fat conscious in the past five years—nutritionists, diet experts, the Surgeon General, and the FDA have cautioned all of us to cut way back on fats and get our cholesterol levels down.

But the incredible health benefit of *lowering protein* is going to take you beyond just losing weight. You'll enhance the function of your heart, liver, kidneys, and immune system. You are going to live longer and better—starting today.

With less protein, you'll be

- saving your body from the ups and downs of fad diets
- saving money because animal protein is the most expensive element in your shopping cart
- saving years off your life

And you'll never have to count calories again. Instead, you'll be counting grams of protein—just 1 gram for every 3 pounds you weigh. I'll show you just what a gram is, and how it fits into the guidelines of the diet. You'll get detailed menu plans, daily charts, and delicious recipes in later chapters.

The Anti-Aging Diet isn't just a weight loss program; it involves a commitment to the future. Your future. This revolutionary plan will not only boost your physical strength and energy, it will forever alter your attitude toward aging.

I think most people expect too little of life. I think we have to develop a burning desire to do more—and for a longer time. And when you feel great today because of the way you're eating, exercising, and developing your potential, you will start to see the added years this diet will give you as a fantastic new set of tools to work with.

Where does modern medical practice fit into the Anti-Aging

Diet? In my twenty-five years in medicine, I've radically changed my beliefs about the role of the physician and the way a doctor can best help his patients.

I believe that medicine of the twenty-first century will be practiced mainly by you—the individual—with your doctor's able assistance. You won't need a doctor to write prescriptions or perform surgery for you, because your newly boosted immune system will keep you healthy without medication or invasive treatment.

In fact, you'll only see your physician once a year, for a complete physical examination. And to find out how he's feeling! If he hasn't made any of the life-style changes that are now part of your life, maybe you can help him get started.

There are, unfortunately, many factors that aren't under our control when it comes to aging. You may live in a stressful, polluted urban environment or have a job that presents a daily risk to your safety. You may not have been blessed with a protective genetic background and may be predisposed to certain cancers or heart disease.

But given all the variables in your particular case, you can still make a difference. Extraordinary documented evidence from the Southwest Health Institute and from laboratories and clinics around the world will prove to you that what you eat does in fact make a significant difference in how healthy you can remain on a day-to-day basis and how much longer—and better—you can live. The low-protein life-style you are about to choose will give you that extra edge.

A certain amount of gradual deterioration does take place as we age that we can't completely stop. But we can slow the process considerably by following the Anti-Aging Diet. Your body, trimmer and leaner from this healthful program, will behave as though it's twenty years younger than your chronological age. Your mind, constantly challenged and receptive to change, will make even more remarkable progress and perform as though you were thirty years younger.

Good Health Can Be Yours

There's no magic pill to ensure good health. But there is a reasonable, easy method! If you want to lose weight, you have to alter your dietary intake and exercise output. If you want to be on top of the hill instead of over the hill, you have to make the commitment and not be afraid to reap the benefits. The amazing thing is that you won't miss any of what you have to give up—damaging proteins, a sedentary life-style, and negative thinking.

Is my Anti-Aging Diet for everyone? Well, I'd say it should be avoided if you've resigned yourself to chronic illness and a fading future. If, on the other hand, you think it's a fabulous idea to feel younger and healthier as you add up those years, if you get a real kick out of people guessing your age as twenty or thirty years younger than you actually are, then it's definitely for you.

Once you're on the Anti-Aging Diet, you'll find you want to stay there for your lifetime because it feels so good. Like a finely tuned automobile, you'll have low-protein, unleaded fuel in your tank that will drive your engine effortlessly. You'll accelerate smoothly and swiftly and coast through your days on a high-energy roll. You'll respond with fingertip ease to situations that once caused you stressful anxiety.

One of my new nurses commented recently that she could always spot people who'd been patients of mine for several years if she met them outside the office. She said that, on average, they seemed to have incredible energy, a better complexion, brighter eyes, and a more positive attitude toward life than most other people she met. I must also add that my patients rarely seem to come down with the common cold and that, no matter their age, many of them testify that their vision and hearing have improved since they've been on the Anti-Aging Diet.

Is this really possible? Of course it is. Each system of the body is intricately related to every other system. The old nutritional cliche, "You are what you eat," may indeed be correct. The less protein damaging the various organs and functions of your body, the greater your overall health.

A Diet that Reverses Disease and Keeps Weight Off

Some physicians who know little about nutrition claim that diet alone cannot make a substantial difference in chronic disease. I beg to differ—and I have the living, breathing, healthy data to prove it. Over the past fifteen years at my Southwest Health Institute, I have implemented the Anti-Aging Diet on 10,000 patients with conditions ranging from heart disease, obesity, kidney disease, arthritis, and gallstones to chronic gastrointestinal problems and early osteoporosis. I can tell you, it works. Over the years, I have seen reversals in disease patterns, weight losses ranging from ten to two hundred pounds, and possible extension of life through my program.

And now you can profit by it, too. If you love life and would like to get more out of it—whether you're 25 or 105—you have everything before you and nothing to lose but unwanted pounds and a pessimistic way of thinking about the future.

In this book, I'll be delighted to share with you not only all the data on the low-protein life-style and the easy and practical application of it to your own life, but also my essential anti-aging truth.

And then, while you're enjoying your extra years, maybe you'll take the time to tell that truth to everyone you know, just to make sure they'll be celebrating their 120th birthday along with you.

Part One

Why the
Anti-Aging Diet?

Chapter 1

The Art of
Growing Younger

How old does the image in your mirror look? More important, how old do you feel when you look at yourself in that mirror? Most days, you probably look your age. Your skin may be a bit sallow or wrinkled, maybe you're picking up a few gray hairs but, overall, the picture you see isn't too bad. Maybe some days you look your age but feel like a kid again. Then there are other times—hopefully few and far between—when you realize that you look and feel decades older than you are—tired and dragged out.

Increasing Your Energy from One Year to the Next

Advertisers love to claim that they can slow the aging process. There are hundreds of products on the market to cover gray, mask wrinkles, and take years off your appearance. But is there really a way to grow younger?

We all know people who have somehow managed to escape the ravages of time: the 49-year-old mother who's often mistaken for her 28-year-old daughter, the 90-year-old great-grandfather who still goes square dancing with his 72-year-old wife twice a week, the 44-year-old lawyer who has the energy to manage a catering service, volunteer for the Red Cross, and perform in a band on weekends.

What magical quality allows them to be so much younger than their years, seeming even more exuberant about life the longer they live it? And where did they get this magic?

Before I answer that question, I have to say that I don't think any of us really want to turn the clock backward. It's not that we'd like to be 18 again and have to bear the slings and arrows of adolescence a second time. I think what we'd probably all like to have is that responsive, athletic body, the amazing ability we used to have to eat and burn every ounce of fat, and maybe, also, the sense of excitement and adventure.

What if you could combine the experience of your years with a very young body? What if you could be flexible, strong and energetic and endowed with the stamina and drive of a much younger person? What if you could slow your own aging process so that by the time you were 50, you'd look and act 30; by the time you're 90, you'd look and act 70?

My Patients Teach Me About Good Health

The Anti-Aging Diet and life-style plan has been honed over years of clinical observation of thousands of patients at my Southwest Health Institute in Phoenix, Arizona. My program has evolved slowly and carefully, and though it's been corroborated by many laboratory trials on protein consumption conducted by well-respected scientists, the Anti-Aging Diet offers a revolutionary new approach to good health.

Feeding rats varying specific amounts of protein in a laboratory setting can suggest what effect eating more or less protein has on humans, but people transcend scientific data. Men and women have minds as well as bodies, emotions, a past, a future—a soul, if you like.

For this reason, I felt that only human beings—my patients—could tell the real story of what was making them healthier and live longer.

And they have. The work I've done with my patients over the last fifteen years—from those who were basically healthy but just a bit overweight and out of shape to those with kidney disease, coronary artery disease, diabetes, chronic obstructive lung disease, arthritis, and osteoporosis—is the real proof.

Scientific validation of a theory often requires trial and error methods, but I did not dare make any mistakes with the men and women who'd entrusted their health and well-being to me. The low-protein strategy I developed and which has helped so many of them to regain health, strength, and joy in life can work for you, as well. This ground-breaking anti-aging program will give you a choice in your ultimate destiny—to have a longer and better life.

On my anti-aging diet, you're going to lose weight and feel better within weeks, and you'll start on the road to growing younger within a few months. You can *and will* make your biological age far younger than your chronological age.

Let me tell you about Janet, a patient of mine. Before she came to see me, she told me at our first appointment, she was forever counting calories, losing a little weight, and then gaining back more than she'd lost. When she wasn't starving herself, she ate too much and in the wrong proportions. She smoked a pack of cigarettes a day and didn't know the meaning of the word exercise.

One of her chief complaints was exhaustion—sometimes she was too tired to get through a full day of work. She was forever reminiscing about her "good years"—her teens and twenties. Only 32 years old, she was certain it was going to be all over for her by the time she'd retired from her job at 65. She imagined the last decades of her life, living out a pitiful existence in a nursing home or being a burden on a younger relative. She was old before her time.

It took Janet six months on the anti-aging program to convince her that her life had just begun. She lost forty pounds, started swimming, and was so filled with energy that her friends told her they didn't recognize her.

Then there was Sam, who at 45 worked professionally to protect the environment, coached T-ball in the evenings, ran or swam every day, and exercised with his wife and son on Sundays. He was a chocolate freak, and he couldn't get through a day without either a steak, a lamb chop, or a pork roast. He was under incredible stress from his job, and his blood pressure was dangerously high. Here was a man who loved life and wanted more of it, but who was also at risk.

I put him on the Anti-Aging Diet with great hopes, because he didn't have an attitude problem. Indeed, my expectations were more than fulfilled. In just three months, his blood pressure had decreased from 170/100 to 120/80, he'd abandoned red meat for grains, legumes and vegetables, and he ate chocolate only on weekends. He had taken up tai ch'i and found that he was able to relax and lower his stress level when he was practicing. When he came back to see me, he told me he loved life even more because he felt so much better about his place in it.

How Old Do You Think You Are?

I think you'll find the following quiz to be a real eye opener because it will direct you to attitudes and behaviors you may not think about often but which bear a direct impact on your ability to grow younger as you age.

Rate yourself from 1 to 3 on each of the following questions. You will find, as you progress on the Anti-Aging Diet, that your score will lower significantly.

Quiz 1. Guessing Your Biological Age

If your score is now from 12 to 16, you are biologically younger than your age.

If you score from 17 to 27, your biological age is the same as your chronological age.

If you score from 28 to 34, you are biologically older than your age.

————— 1. How old do you feel?
    Younger than your age   Add 1
    Your chronological age   2
    Older than your age   3

————— 2. How does your skin appear? (Do you have wrinkling and sagging—some, or none?)
    Excellent   1
    Average   2
    Poor   3

————— 3. How is your posture?
    Erect   1
    Average   2
    Stooped   3

————— 4. How flexible is your body?
    You can put your leg on a kitchen counter and touch your toe   1
    You can put your leg on the counter, but you can't touch your toe   2
    You can't get your leg on the counter   3

————— 5. How is your weight?
    Within five pounds of ideal weight   1
    Need to lose ten to twenty pounds   2
    Need to lose more than twenty pounds   3

————— 6. What's your general mental attitude?
    Positive   1
    Mixed   2
    Negative   3

_____ 7. Are you physically fit?

     You can walk more than 3 miles without difficulty   1

     You can walk more than a mile without difficulty   2

     You're unable to walk a mile   3

_____ 8. Do you suffer from chronic disease?

     You've been medically diagnosed as healthy   1

     You've been medically diagnosed as having either hypertension or diabetes   2

     You've been medically diagnosed as having either heart or lung disease or cancer other than skin cancer   3

_____ 9. How much regular medication do you take?

     None   1

     One   2

     Two or more   3

_____ 10. What is your activity level?

     Work full-time (paid or volunteer position)   1

     Work part-time   2

     Housewife or househusband   3

_____ 11. What is your energy level?

     High all day until you go to sleep at night   1

     High all day until you come home from work   2

     Energy low by 2:00 P.M.   3

_____ 12. What is your level of sexual activity in a monogamous relationship?

     Twice or more weekly   1

     Once a week   2

     Once a month   3

_____ TOTAL

Why Americans Age Faster Than Other People

The leading causes of death in our country for people over 65 are heart disease, cancer, stroke, diabetes, influenza and pneumonia, arteriosclerosis, and accidents, in descending order of frequency. After these are emphysema and asthma, liver cirrhosis, and kidney failure.

You're probably thinking, well, I'm too young to have any of those diseases. I might get hit by a car or drown in the bathtub, but I'm certainly not susceptible to cancer or a heart attack—not yet. In fact, statistics show that your age has nothing to do with whether you're prone to serious illness. Instead, what does matter is your resistance factor and the ability of your cells to repair themselves.

Take pneumonia as a classic case. We all know somebody over 65 who fell and broke her hip and was taken to the hospital where she contracted pneumonia and died. Did she succumb to the pneumonia because of a broken bone or because her immune system response was lowered? Was her immune system affected by the stress of being ill and away from home? Maybe she had the bad luck to have a genetic predisposition to osteoporosis or brittle bones, and her hip broke before she fell.

Which is it? It's really impossible to say. There's a little environment and a little genetic input in everything that goes on in the body. We can't do anything about our genes, but we can make a real difference in our susceptibility to disease.

The best protection is *prevention*. The better care you can take of your internal organs, the longer they'll function at peak performance. That means, the stronger you are, the better your resistance—regardless of age.

The Chinese, the Georgians formerly of the Soviet Union, the Fiji Islanders, and dozens of other groups contract fewer life-threatening diseases and age more slowly than Americans. Our medical technology is by far the most advanced but our preventive approaches are by far the worst.

What are we doing wrong that they're doing right? A variety of things, but I'll give you one major clue: They eat one-half to one-third the amount of protein we do.

We fortunate Americans have too much food—most of it processed—and, in general, it's eaten on the run because we're all so busy. Most Americans tend to grab a frozen meal or something in a package that was created in a laboratory for high-efficiency ease of preparation. Most people drive a car to work, sit at a desk all day, and then sit in front of the television several hours every evening.

More than any other culture on earth, we are systematically killing ourselves with excess. Despite the world's most advanced medical technology, we suffer from the diseases of affluence: heart conditions and obesity from the wrong kind of eating, lung diseases from smoking, osteoporosis, and lessened physical endurance from lack of activity. It doesn't have to stay that way, though. By following my anti-aging diet, you will turn excess into variety; you'll grow younger as you grow older. By eating, exercising, and thinking differently, you will effectively change your expectations for the way you feel today, tomorrow, and for the rest of your life.

What Promotes Long Life?

I've always been fascinated by cultures where extreme longevity is the norm. Only several hundred miles from my home in Phoenix, the Tarahumara Indians of northern Mexico routinely live for over a hundred years. So do peasants in the Russian Caucasus and in many mainland Chinese villages. Why is this? What do they have that we don't, what do they do that allows them to stretch their life span and avoid most diseases of modern civilization?

- People tend to eat less, in great part because there is less to eat
- People usually live in extended family situations, thus eliminating the loneliness and depression that tends to come with age in our society

- People are expected to work hard and be active as long as they're alive
- People don't call themselves old, but "honorable" or "venerable" when they pass 80; others don't think of them as old but as repositories of wisdom and experience
- People have an expected routine to their days. Without access to fast-track living, they never even experience jet lag, because they don't have to go anywhere. They never have the problem of their company transferring them after a few years in one location. The workplace, home, and center of leisure activities tend to be within walking distance of each other

These differences are significant, because they touch on the society's image of aging. Stereotypes about the worth of living longer can't be changed overnight. However, as you alter your own perception of aging well and start getting rid of some ingrained habits, you'll see that a desire for good health can be catching. We'll all want to lower our biological age if we can look and feel the way you do.

Mind and Body as One Healthy Unit

Just like the body, the mind and emotions are also susceptible to coming down with something. I'm not talking about a specific mental illness like schizophrenia or Alzheimer's, which strike only a small segment of our society. I'm talking about the kind of attitude that stops you from getting ahead, getting well, or living better.

Positive mental attitude enhances your resistance to physical disease. We can take the case of the strange Epstein-Barr virus, which often attacks young, fast-track people who have high stress levels, paralyzing them with chronic fatigue. As it happens, 90 percent of the population actually has Epstein-Barr antibodies present in their system, but 90 percent of the population doesn't get the disease.

Those who do succumb to it are frequently people who are depressed; being depressed, they're often unable to handle stress, which makes them more susceptible to the condition.

It is found, increasingly, that those people who can snap back from a debilitating illness or crippling accident are those with a powerful self-healing spirit that surpasses all physical odds. There are documented cases of many individuals close to death who have somehow been able to muster the will to survive despite all their doctors' predictions. They are examples of mind-fitness immunization—and an inspiration to us all.

Mind Fitness

The human body is in a constant state of flux, but so is the human mind. And it's here that the most interesting part of aging—or not aging—goes on.

Quiz 2. How Fit Is Your Mind?

Each "true" answer earns you a point. The closer you come to a score of 12, the fitter your mind is.

If you score 7 to 12 points, your mind is fabulously fit.

If you score 4 to 6 points, you need to make some changes in your diet, exercise, and mind fitness.

If you score 0 to 3 points, you need to seek an emotional support system, i.e., professional counseling, meditation tapes or classes, or biofeedback counseling.

_____ 1. You never take medication, i.e., tranquilizers, sleeping pills, or recreational drugs, to relieve stress
_____ 2. You never smoke or drink alcohol
_____ 3. You never eat compulsively
_____ 4. You never lose emotional control and act in a hostile manner toward others
_____ 5. You never "blank out" i.e., go to sleep or watch TV—and deny your feelings

————— 6. You exercise in order to reduce stress
————— 7. You meditate or spend some time alone
————— 8. You let go of the problem and go on with your life
————— 9. You laugh and have fun
————— 10. You look forward to the future
————— 11. Instead of warring with yourself, you make love with someone else
————— 12. You see yourself, happy and healthy, at 120

————————— TOTAL

Slowing the Aging Process

So how are we going to combine the benefits of our high-tech, fast-paced American life-style with the protective elements of a simpler life? How can we slow the aging process?

When I was a kid growing up in Philadelphia, I used to hear my elderly relatives say, "You've got nothing unless you've got your health." They were absolutely right.

Unfortunately, most of them did nothing to correct the old bad habits of ill health they'd been practicing for years. They thought it was luck—either you had good health or you didn't.

I say that although there's a certain amount of luck involved—you can be born with a terrific set of genes or a set you'd prefer to send back for alterations—ultimately, you have to take charge. You have to make a major investment in your health now.

The first thing you're going to do to increase your assets, oddly enough, is make a withdrawal. You're going to take a whopping amount of protein out of your diet. Then you'll start making your deposits, adding in other nutritional factors, a modest amount of exercise, and a positive attitude. You'll draw on those deposits occasionally (when you catch a cold, for example), and then you'll get to reinvest them. But oh, the dividends you're going to reap as you get older!

Another Step Toward Living Longer

I'd like you to work through the following profile to open your health account today. In it, you can assess your potential for long life, or detect the harmful elements you can reduce or eliminate in order to increase your longevity. Add to or subtract from your starting age as indicated. The bottom line is how long you can live.

Quiz 3. Longevity Profile

If you are a man, start with 72, which is the current average male life expectancy.

If you are a woman, start with 78, which is the current average female life expectancy.

_____ 1. CURRENT AGE
Your life expectancy increases the older you are. Women initially have an extra edge on men because naturally occurring estrogens give them protection against heart disease. After menopause, at about age 50, as estrogen levels decline, the odds even out.

FOR MEN	FOR WOMEN
If you're 20 to 30, add 1	If you're 20 to 30, add 5
If you're 30 to 40, add 2	If you're 30 to 40, add 6
If you're 40 to 50, add 3	If you're 40 to 50, add 7
If you're 50 to 60, add 4	If you're 50 to 60, add 4
If you're 60 to 70, add 5	If you're 60 to 70, add 5
If you're over 70, add 6	If you're over 70, add 6

_____ 2. WEIGHT
If you're within five pounds of your ideal weight, add 5
If you're five to ten pounds overweight, subtract 1
If you're ten to twenty pounds overweight, subtract 2
If you're twenty to thirty pounds overweight, subtract 3
If you're thirty to fifty pounds overweight, subtract 5
If you're more than fifty pounds overweight, subtract 7

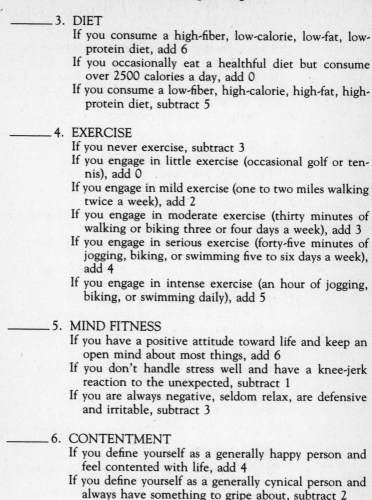

_____ 3. DIET

If you consume a high-fiber, low-calorie, low-fat, low-protein diet, add 6

If you occasionally eat a healthful diet but consume over 2500 calories a day, add 0

If you consume a low-fiber, high-calorie, high-fat, high-protein diet, subtract 5

_____ 4. EXERCISE

If you never exercise, subtract 3

If you engage in little exercise (occasional golf or tennis), add 0

If you engage in mild exercise (one to two miles walking twice a week), add 2

If you engage in moderate exercise (thirty minutes of walking or biking three or four days a week), add 3

If you engage in serious exercise (forty-five minutes of jogging, biking, or swimming five to six days a week), add 4

If you engage in intense exercise (an hour of jogging, biking, or swimming daily), add 5

_____ 5. MIND FITNESS

If you have a positive attitude toward life and keep an open mind about most things, add 6

If you don't handle stress well and have a knee-jerk reaction to the unexpected, subtract 1

If you are always negative, seldom relax, are defensive and irritable, subtract 3

_____ 6. CONTENTMENT

If you define yourself as a generally happy person and feel contented with life, add 4

If you define yourself as a generally cynical person and always have something to gripe about, subtract 2

_____ 7. AUTOMOBILE SAFETY

If you always wear a seatbelt and have no violations, add 3

If you've had any minor violations in the past year, subtract 1

If you've had one or more accidents in the past year, subtract 2

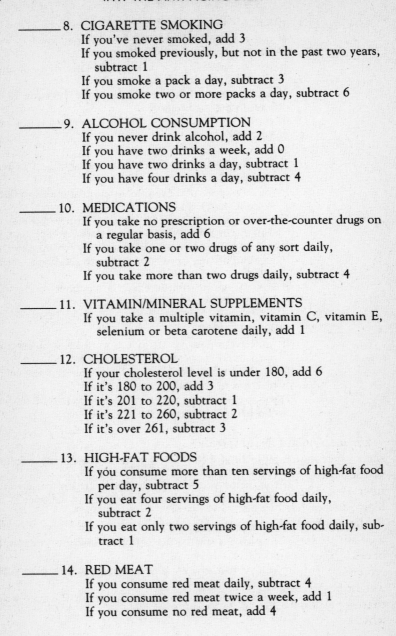

_____ 8. CIGARETTE SMOKING

If you've never smoked, add 3

If you smoked previously, but not in the past two years, subtract 1

If you smoke a pack a day, subtract 3

If you smoke two or more packs a day, subtract 6

_____ 9. ALCOHOL CONSUMPTION

If you never drink alcohol, add 2

If you have two drinks a week, add 0

If you have two drinks a day, subtract 1

If you have four drinks a day, subtract 4

_____ 10. MEDICATIONS

If you take no prescription or over-the-counter drugs on a regular basis, add 6

If you take one or two drugs of any sort daily, subtract 2

If you take more than two drugs daily, subtract 4

_____ 11. VITAMIN/MINERAL SUPPLEMENTS

If you take a multiple vitamin, vitamin C, vitamin E, selenium or beta carotene daily, add 1

_____ 12. CHOLESTEROL

If your cholesterol level is under 180, add 6

If it's 180 to 200, add 3

If it's 201 to 220, subtract 1

If it's 221 to 260, subtract 2

If it's over 261, subtract 3

_____ 13. HIGH-FAT FOODS

If you consume more than ten servings of high-fat food per day, subtract 5

If you eat four servings of high-fat food daily, subtract 2

If you eat only two servings of high-fat food daily, subtract 1

_____ 14. RED MEAT

If you consume red meat daily, subtract 4

If you consume red meat twice a week, add 1

If you consume no red meat, add 4

_____ 13. EDUCATIONAL LEVEL
   If you are a male college graduate, add 2
   If you are a female college graduate, add 5

_____ 14. PARENTAL LONGEVITY
   If your father is still living and is older than 75, add 2
   If your father died before age 75, add 0
   If your father died before age sixty, subtract 2
   If your father died before age fifty, subtract 4

_____ 15. CHRONIC DISEASE
   (Various disease states will not necessarily affect physi-
      ological aging, but they can have a significant impact
      on your longevity.)
   If you do not suffer from hypertension, diabetes, heart
      disease, lung disease, or cancer, add 5
   If you've been medically diagnosed as having
      —hypertension, subtract 3
      —diabetes, subtract 4
      —heart disease, subtract 5
      —lung disease, subtract 6
      —cancer (except benign skin cancer), subtract 10

_____ TOTAL

Betting on Wellness

Let me tell you about a truly remarkable patient of mine. She's
such a terrific example of the life-changing and life-giving portion
of the Anti-Aging Diet that I am constantly inspired by her. Jennifer is a 30-year-old school teacher, and the eloquent lesson I
learned from her has been invaluable in my practice.

She weighed 340 pounds when she first came to see me. At five
feet six inches tall, she fell into the category called "morbidly
obese." She'd been overweight for so many years, she couldn't ever
remember being normal. She told me she'd never tried to lose
weight before, that her "earth suit," as she called it, had not been
that important to her. But now it was, although she wouldn't say
why.

She lost 22 pounds during the first week of the Anti-Aging Diet—more initial weight loss than any of my previous patients at the Southwest Health Institute. During the first month, she lost over 50 pounds.

I quizzed her thoroughly to make sure she was really eating all the food she was supposed to consume, and she assured me that she was eating heartily—but it was the exercise part of the diet that had facilitated the remarkable weight loss.

Okay, let's cut to the chase. After two years with me, she'd lost 200 pounds; she looked and felt wonderful. The following statistics on Jennifer are just the shallow indications of what really was happening to her mind and body:

	Initially	*Two Years Later*
cholesterol	400	150
blood pressure	180/100	110/70
weight	340	140
kidney function	BUN 22	BUN 15

But what is more remarkable than these clinical changes is the fact that Jennifer was betting on wellness; she was looking for a future. At the end of two years, she finally told me what her motivation had been.

She had lost the weight for her father who was dying of cancer and had asked for just one thing—that she not compromise her health in any way. She told me that her feelings of mortality had been so heightened during the time that her father was sick that she knew she could never end up like him—in a hospital bed, attached to machines, eventually too weak and debilitated to want to live another day.

But she did more than survive. She changed her life. And I know that she will never turn back.

The health care and insurance industries have grown enormously in the past decade. They're betting that Americans are going to live longer but will become ill—perhaps even incapacitated—by the time they reach the upper limits of their life span.

But there's nothing sicker than the American health care system. It's probably going to suffer cardiac arrest and require a heart transplant in the twenty-first century. This incredibly complex system with all the high-tech medical wizardry behind it simply can't survive much longer in its present form because it can't continue to pay for itself. No one will be able to afford the premiums they'd have to pay to get well. The only alternative, as I see it, is never to become sick enough to have to use the system.

Even if your health benefits are paid for by your employer, you must be acutely aware of how much of your monthly paycheck now goes to medical insurance. You can never get back the money your insurance allocates for illnesses you don't have yet but might have in the future. There is even an option offered by many major corporations that allows employees to contribute up to $5,000 annually to a tax-free plan, something like an IRA or Keogh, that can only be used to pay for medical bills. If you don't get sick, you lose all that money!

Life insurance is another industry that bets on your getting sick. Term life insurance becomes more expensive the older you get. If you live well into your nineties, you probably won't be able to afford the premiums. Some whole life plans have a cut-off date. If you haven't died by that time, you're cancelled.

My feeling is that the powers that be are growing increasingly concerned about how long everyone is going to live. They are working under the assumption that high-tech medicine simply won't be enough, and that by the year 2020, we're going to be a nation overrun with invalid, senile elderly who need chronic care.

But what if we, like my inspirational patient Jennifer, can change that thinking by taking steps now to remain healthy so that we grow stronger instead of weaker over time? What if we bank on wellness? I'm not saying you should stop paying your insurance premiums, but I am saying that I want you to start thinking differently about the way you're going to age once you're on my anti-aging diet.

If you pay attention to my simple guidelines, you're naturally going to grow younger biologically, no matter what your chronological age, starting right now.

Chapter 2

The Search for a Revolutionary Diet

What I have to say about protein is definitely going to shock you: You're eating too much of it. As a matter of fact, if you're a typical American man or woman between the ages of 25 and 65, you could cut your protein intake by half and be much healthier. And, perhaps even more importantly, you would slow down your aging process.

I know this contradicts everything you've ever heard about protein. But I told you you'd have to be open-minded when you approached this radical new way to eat and to live. The Anti-Aging Diet is going to shatter a myth that has prevailed for the last fifty years—that the more protein you eat, the more energetic, stronger, and better you'll feel. The opposite is true! You are in fact slowing yourself down, wearing yourself out, and aging yourself prematurely by eating more protein.

I developed my life-style diet for my patients at the Southwest Health Institute because I saw that they were going to have different physical, mental, and emotional needs than the last generation had. Our parents didn't have to worry about feeling 40 at 65 or living to 100; the only thing most of them were looking forward to was retirement.

We, on the other hand, are the first individuals in history with the potential to consider *active longevity*. I don't mean at some vague point in the future, but right away. My goal is to start you in your thirties and forties on a protective, preventive, challenging program that will give you the will and the way to do more now than you ever have and continue with undiminished forces to a very advanced age.

The Wrong Food;
The Right Intention

Eating less protein is going to unlock that door for you. Allow me to explain.

I used to eat as though my internal organs and my mouth were in two separate bodies. I ate because I was hungry, because food tasted good, because I needed energy to keep going at the frenetic pace that has been my pattern since I was a kid in Philadelphia.

My first exposure to food, of course, was at home. My Jewish mother spent days slaving over traditional foods that were high in fat (chicken soup with dumplings made with *schmaltz*, or rendered chicken fat), high in fat and sugar (egg-based breads and cakes with lots of sugar and jam), and off the scale in protein (brisket of beef, boiled chicken, lamb, herring, and so on).

Also, I was a real Philly kid, which meant that after school I'd indulge in Philly cheese steaks, pizza, hoagies (also known as submarines), and soft pretzels covered with salt and dipped in mustard. I was a nutritional mess—but I didn't know it!

I had never run a mile before my last year in medical school. But one day, feeling like I had to get away from the books for a while, I tried it and liked it. Running seemed to refresh my mind and body and make it easier for me to study effectively. After a couple of years of running for my health, I got competitive about it and decided I wanted to improve my running times. After doing some interesting reading about athletes' diets, I decided to experiment with my own. And it was then that I began to realize that everything I'd ever learned about eating was wrong.

A Brief History of Diets

In every era, there have been those who declare that one particular type of diet is a panacea. Originally, nutritionists believed that you only had to reduce calories to lose—you had to starve yourself on lettuce and fruit salad and cottage cheese, maybe just a bit of boiled chicken or fish for dinner. After you cut out anything delicious like pasta or dessert and you'd faithfully consumed only 800 to 1000 calories a day for three weeks, there you were—ravenous, but thinner. There's a simple formula based on calories that goes like this:

- When you take in fewer calories than you expend, you lose weight
- When you take in more calories than you expend, you gain weight

But calories are only one factor in the great weight plan. The human body is far too complicated for something as simple as this formula to work for everyone all the time. The biochemistry of each individual depends on many factors, such as thermogenesis, basal metabolism, setpoint, and genetics, to name just a few. The reason that so many diets of the '60s and '70s fell by the wayside was that pounds shed by drastically reducing caloric intake were invariably gained right back as soon as you stopped eating in this unpleasant, artificial manner and began to eat regular meals again.

Then came the high-protein diets—steak and boiled eggs or lamb chops and cheese sauce, all washed down with lots of water. Dr. Atkins, who originally touted this diet in 1973,[1] was part of a long tradition that began back in the 1890s, when the USDA recommended 110 grams of dietary protein per day for working men. (Just compare this to my recommendation, which is 60 grams for a 180-pound man!)

Here's how the high-protein concept works: When you eat protein, it's converted into amino acids to meet your body's requirements for maintenance and repair. Any amino acids left over are then either converted to glycogen in the liver or stored as fat, and then your body gets rid of the excess nitrogen created when protein is converted to fat or glycogen.

To supply your energy needs, your body first burns the carbohydrates you eat. If your body has completely depleted its carbohydrate stores, it will start to burn the protein and fat that would otherwise be used for cell repair, metabolism, and energy storage. This is the situation when the body is deprived of carbohydrates for long periods of time, if you're starving to death on a desert island, for example.

The diet books that touted high protein a few decades ago, beginning with Dr. Atkins's, worked on the theory that if the body had no carbohydrates or fat, nothing but protein to utilize for energy, it would eat up its own fat and tissue and you'd lose weight. A great deal of water would be necessary to break down the fat and protein and then excrete the wastes, but you were supposed to drink enormous quantities of water to compensate for the loss.

When you metabolize protein this way, you lose nitrogen through your urine and sweat. Nitrogen, a gas that exists in the atmosphere and in all living things, is essential for tissue building. We get our nitrogen from the protein in our systems and the protein we eat. Then we break down that protein in the liver and kidneys. Finally we excrete nitrogen through our urine, sweat, and feces. Nitrogen balance is crucial to the body. The less protein in your diet, the less excess nitrogen you have to excrete. The more protein in your diet, the more excess nitrogen you have to excrete, the result being a nitrogen imbalance and more work for your liver and kidneys. It's all right to be in this state for six miles or an hour of intensive marathon running, but it is very unhealthy to be in this state for the duration of most diets. The high-protein diets did take weight off but were unsafe because they caused nitrogen imbalance, which left the dieters feeling weak and listless. And the weight was regained as soon as you added carbohydrates to your menus and shifted the dangerous nitrogen imbalance back to normal.

In the 1980s, a variety of diet doctors came out with what I call the high-carbohydrate single-food diets. They understood correctly that the body burns carbohydrates quickly as fuel; what they did not take into account was that variety is essential for this process to work properly. So there was a rice diet and a fruit diet and a diet where you had to eat lentil soup for breakfast, potatoes for lunch, and pasta with nothing on it for dinner. The complexity of these plans was supposed to trick the body into burning different amino acids at different times. All it really did was, once again, make people eat in ways that were antithetical to real life consumption. Once the weight was lost and they went back to old patterns, they gained again.

As medical science learned more about dietary fat, we were bombarded with articles and books about low-fat eating. It has been conclusively proven in laboratory and human studies that cutting the amount of saturated fat in the diet can reduce your risk of heart disease and stroke, lower blood pressure, and take off weight. Americans are more aware of health risks today than they were ten years ago, thanks to the information now accessible to all. However, they still don't heed most of the advice given by experts about fat in the diet.

But I had an inkling of an idea that went beyond healthy hearts and weight loss. I wanted to be in great shape in my marathoning days—but I also wanted to find out more about what kinds of foods would keep me in this kind of shape for the rest of my life. My eventual goal was to create a lifetime program that would make me and my patients as healthy and fit at 90 or 100 as at 30. But until I had all the pieces of the puzzle in place, I wasn't about to experiment with anyone but myself.

I love to eat and would have gone batty on a limited diet. I couldn't count calories (who has the inclination to do something so time consuming that nets you absolutely nothing?). I wanted to develop a way of eating a very large number of varied foods that would provide the most nutrients and give me the greatest energy expenditure per gram of food ingested.

A Radical New Thought: Less Protein Is More

In 1904, Dr. R. H. Chittenden, a physiologist at Yale University, studied twenty-four healthy male subjects over long periods of time in various states of activity. This amazing researcher, light-years ahead of his time, demonstrated that adults would thrive eating a low-protein diet: subjects consumed only about 55 grams of protein a day, a level about half that of the standard of the day, which was 118 to 125 grams.[2]

He also discovered that the athletes in his group were able to increase their strength and speed performance. The improvements he noted in fifteen strength tests over a six-month period on a low-protein diet simply go off the scale! The total strength measurements for all the men at least doubled and, in some cases, tripled. He theorized that a low-protein diet allows more energy expenditure per gram of food intake than a high-protein diet. And thermogenesis, the ability of the body to burn calories efficiently, was enhanced on a low-protein diet. In effect, the athletes could eat more and gain less.

But no one I knew or studied in medical school ever quoted Chittenden. As a matter of fact, his theory was considered outrageous. Everyone I knew in the nutrition and fitness fields said that high-protein eating was essential for athletes. Remember all those guys on the football teams chowing down on steaks and chops just before a game? Dr. Atkins had popularized the longstanding myth of high-protein eating, and many respected nutritionists and physicians had followed in his footsteps. Who was I to start knocking protein?

Why I Reduced My Protein Consumption

One of the earliest researchers of the aging process was Dr. Clive McCay at Cornell University.[3] I was reading about his studies just before I ran my first marathon in 1971. A pioneer in 1939, he divided rats into different groups and at first tried giving them smaller amounts of a regular, well-balanced diet—a diet in which 20 percent of the calories come from protein. This percentage is generally considered sufficient to allow a laboratory animal to grow and develop normally.

Though his underfed animals were small, they all lived long after the rats fed the normal diet had died. In later experiments, he underfed the animals and also decreased the amount of protein in the diet. The rats fed less protein lived longest of all, and their low-protein diet kept them 25 to 30 percent thinner than the animals on the diet with the regular amount of protein. The rats fed less protein had coats that were smooth and shiny. They also developed far fewer cancers than the high-protein rats.[4]

I ran my first marathon in 4 hours and 7 minutes. I wanted to do better, and I knew I could. I hadn't given up on protein—I felt there was just too much data indicating that athletes needed it— but I thought perhaps changing the balance of my eating might make a difference.

I was also influenced by the work of Drs. Bergstrom and Hultman and Ahlborg in Scandinavia. In 1967, they had published some extraordinary data on carbohydrate loading and depletion, and the evidence seemed so convincing, I decided to try it for my next marathon.[5]

Prior to serious physical exertion, they said, an athlete should consume a total protein diet for three days, then load up on pasta, cereals, breads, vegetables, and fruits for three days, then compete. Though the Swedish doctors' studies were on cycling rather than running, I figured the results would still apply to me.

The Principle of Carbohydrate Depletion

The body's need for protein fluctuates daily, even hourly. When you're sitting in a chair, reading, you don't need very much at all; when you're injured or going through a very stressful event, your need can increase significantly. But the body can perform some amazing balancing acts. Without your doing anything at all, it can call on your protein reserves to take care of difficult physical or psychological stress.

A marathoner is going to be under acute physical stress for several hours. The theory was that by depleting carbohydrates for three days and then loading carbohydrates for the next three, you would be forcing the body to make the best use of its energy stores. When you eat only protein, you deplete the muscle cells of glycogen and deny the liver its ability to store glycogen for three days. You are, in a sense, opening the cells up so they can hold more glycogen on the three days of carbohydrate loading just prior to the race.

Why Protein Loading
Doesn't Work

I realized during my three days on carbohydrate depletion that something was radically wrong. When I ate only meals high in animal protein and no carbohydrates, I felt weaker, more irritable, and more lethargic than I had ever felt in my life. The reason: I was overloading on amino acids, I developed nitrogen imbalance, and my body reacted violently.

Then a work on the Eskimo diet, done in 1974 by Mazess and Mather, came to my attention.[6] This conclusive study was done on the bone mineral content of Eskimos, who ate virtually nothing but animal protein—sea mammals, caribou, fish, and birds were the staples of their diet. Eskimos over the age of 40 had about 10 to 15 percent less bone density than those of whites of the same age. Their rate of bone loss was about 2 to 3 percent a year per decade. The reason for this loss is that a meat diet, high in amino acids, has an acidic effect on the blood and increases the excretion of calcium through the urine. Studies have shown that when people consume more than 100 grams of protein a day, they develop a negative calcium balance. This means that their calcium levels start to decrease (as in the case of the Eskimos) and osteoporosis, a disease where the bones become weaker and prone to breakage, becomes a real threat.

Why does a high meat diet have such a deleterious effect on the bones? In order to understand this, you must know that the blood needs to be kept at an even PH balance. During the breakdown of protein, a negative charge occurs in the blood and it becomes acidic—its PH lowers. The electrolytes (all the minerals in the body such as calcium, potassium, magnesium, and sodium), which carry a positive charge, must suddenly rush to the rescue. In order to reduce that acidic effect of the amino acid breakdown, the minerals leach out of the bones to balance the PH of the blood.

As I learned, athletes should be consuming average amounts of dietary protein and vitamins if they're interested in extra energy. Too much protein is harmful to the kidneys and liver and will tear down—not build up—the body's systems. You may remember that when anabolic steroids fell into disrepute, many body builders started taking supplemental amino acids that were touted by advertisers as muscle-building aids. Athletes have been fed a lot of ridiculous misinformation about protein powder, which has been claimed by some to be the power food for enhanced performance.

And, unfortunately, if they continue gobbling extra amino acids or power protein drinks, they may find to their dismay that they're actually becoming weaker, not stronger. Over time, excess dietary protein will destroy their bones, kidneys, and liver.

Another Piece in the Low-Protein Puzzle

After consuming only protein for three days, my program required me to eat only complex carbohydrates for the next three days, just prior to the race. What an extraordinary difference I felt! With very little protein, my energy soared, my legs filled with strength, and my mind was clear. I felt as though I could take on the world. And I did finish that marathon in 3 hours 30 minutes: my times were coming down.

Yet I felt that this success was due only to the carbohydrate-loading schedule right before the race; I'd nearly killed myself with three days of animal protein. My own experience had convinced me, and it has since been documented, that carbohydrate depletion is potentially detrimental to athletes. Clyde Williams, in the *American Journal of Clinical Nutrition*, writes, "There are doubts, however, about the advisability of including the low-carbohydrate phase in the dietary and exercise manipulation procedure. Not only is it a very unpleasant period, which undermines the confidence of the athlete at a time when he is preparing for competition, but there is the real fear of exercise-induced hypoglycemia during the 3 [days] on the low-carbohydrate diet."[7]

I completely agree. So for the next year I cut out animal protein almost entirely—no red meat, chicken, or fish. I still ate some cheese and drank some milk, but most of my protein came from plant sources—legumes and vegetables.

That year, I didn't have a cold, I never had a stomachache. I had always been highly allergic at various times of the year, but I found that year that my symptoms were far milder than in previous years. Although my seasonal allergies hadn't vanished, I didn't need and didn't take any medication, and I was just fine. When the Hong Kong flu laid all my colleagues and friends low, it just passed me by. I kept training and working hard. I had boundless energy. Although I didn't understand this at the time, recent research has explained the results.

Dr. Ronda Bell, of Cornell University, working in the laboratory of Dr. T. Colin Campbell, has done some fascinating work on the way that low-protein diets affect immune surveillance in the body.[8] For thirteen months, she kept some rats on a 22-percent protein diet and others on a 6-percent protein diet. She injected them all with carcinogens that attack the liver. The amazing results were that the rats fed the low-protein diet had an enhanced production of natural killer (or NK) cells that roam the body and destroy cancerous cells. The rats on the low-protein diet stayed cancer free and lived longer than their colleagues fed more protein.

Evidently, like the rats, I was healthier in general because my immune surveillance was up.

The low-protein concept began to crystallize for me. Not only did eating less protein make me feel better, I really *was* better. My immune system functioned at its peak, my liver and kidneys weren't overly taxed, and my bones were calcium rich.

But Does It Work? It Does!

I started getting stronger and was now lifting weights, bench pressing over two hundred pounds, doing four sets of twenty repetitions per set on several different machines (the equivalent of working out with over ten thousand pounds of weight per workout). I was astonished at how fast I improved.

My next marathon, I decided, would really be my turning point. If a low-protein diet was truly a breakthrough in nutritional science, if I was the first guinea pig (beyond all those healthy rats, of course!) and the diet worked, I would do some more medical investigation and see how I could make the diet a part of my patients' regimens.

Voilà! I ran the Boston Marathon of 1978 in 3 hours and 21 minutes, breaking my previous best time by nine minutes. Having already cut nearly an hour from my marathon time, I had been convinced I couldn't get any faster. And yet, here I was, down another 20 seconds per mile. The low-protein experiment had worked brilliantly. But I still had some research to do before I told the world about it.

Chapter 3

The Overrated Protein

Everyone's been telling you for years that protein is good. Meat and milk and eggs have probably been staples of your diet since you were a child, but today's the day you're going to change all that.

Protein stresses all the body's organs in one way or another; various studies have shown that a high-protein diet is often implicated in diabetes, heart disease, cancer, ulcers, strokes, and gouty arthritis. By reducing your protein intake, you can completely change the prognosis for wear and tear over the years. Your body will not only look fitter externally, it will be stronger internally and far more resistant to disease once you reverse the balance of what you eat.

Before I tell you about the many ways in which a low-protein diet is going to completely change what's in store for you today, and for many years to come, I must stop a moment and go over the basics about the relative importance of protein in the body because the evidence will prove to you conclusively that my Anti-Aging Diet is going to work for you.

Each human being is an amazing amalgam of chemicals that react and interact in specific ways to keep you healthy and functional. You may not be aware that over half of you is made up of water—women are 55 percent and men are 60 percent water. Half of the remaining percentage is protein, a protein made up of building blocks known as amino acids.

Protein is responsible for structure in your body: hair, skin, nails, cartilage, muscle, and bone are all mostly protein. Your body also uses protein for metabolism; some hormones and all enzymes are protein, too. Your red blood cells, which carry oxygen, are made of protein. Protein also helps regulate water balance and the acid/alkaline balance in the body. If you didn't have protein, you couldn't generate antibodies to protect yourself against disease.

Amino Acids: The Building Blocks of Protein

There are twenty-two amino acids that build protein molecules, and eight of these—known as the essential amino acids—can't be manufactured by the human body. L-tryptophan, leucine, isoleucine, lysine, valine, threonine, phenylalanine, the sulphurated amino acid methionine, and cystine must be absorbed from what you eat, from what's known as your dietary protein. Once you've consumed these eight from the foods in your diet, your body can make the rest.

The important thing about protein is not how much you take in, but how much your body really needs. If you eat more protein than your body needs, the excess will not be stored as protein; it will be converted to fat.

Amino acids are *reusable*. As protein is broken down in the body, some of it is used for structural work and some is used for metabolic work. Some protein is recycled and used to form other proteins later on, when and where the body needs it. If the protein level in the body rises, the liver will store the extra amino acids for a limited time until the level goes down. At this point, the liver can send the stores back into circulation again. Other cells in the body can store amino acids, too. According to Arthur C. Guyton, author of *The Physiology of the Body*, this amino acid pool insures that the body can always recycle its proteins. Guyton's work conclusively proved that a human being can function perfectly well for thirty days without any animal or vegetable protein at all.[1]

But if too much dietary protein is consumed, nitrogen will be excreted as waste matter. Excess protein and amino acids are degraded in the liver and the waste is sent to the kidneys for elimination. The more work the kidneys and liver have to do to process the waste, the more stress is placed on these organs.

When you eat less protein than your body is used to getting, however, your protein synthesis and breakdown become more efficient. Fewer amino acids are broken down, and there is less stress on your kidneys and liver. The body adjusts and compensates and becomes a better functioning machine.

Animal Protein versus Vegetable Protein

There are two types of protein: animal and vegetable. Animal protein comes from eggs, cheese, milk, meat, and chicken—probably the current staples of your diet. But when you eat protein that comes from animal sources, you're also eating a great deal of saturated fat and cholesterol. This is a costly risk to take because it's much harder for your body to process this type of protein, and the saturated fat that you take in along with it is a clear health danger, since it collects on arterial walls—particularly those of your heart—and forms plaque deposits that inhibit blood flow.

Think about the last time you ate a Big Mac or a twelve-ounce steak from the grill. Did you just feel comfortably satiated, or did you feel overly full for several hours afterward? I bet you felt stuffed.

You felt stuffed because the animal protein works its way very slowly through your digestive system, and your gastrointestinal tract is full hours after eating. You're using more of what you've eaten for energy because it takes your body longer to metabolize animal protein. The reason for this is that animal protein is loaded with fat, which is the most difficult element the body has to digest. Fat is a more complex food than protein or carbohydrate and is more difficult to break down and digest. The digestive tract itself slows down in order to accommodate fats—even producing the enzymes that digest fat takes longer. You feel logy, fatigued, and sometimes constipated owing to the slowing down of your digestive process. And this slow digestion increases the amount of time that potentially carcinogenic food agents can come in contact with your bowel, causing you to be more susceptible to colon cancer.

Typically, it takes a steak about 16 hours to be metabolized by your body and make it through your digestive system. On the other hand, a high-fiber carbohydrate with all the vegetable protein you need, like pasta, takes only 8 hours. That means fast utilization of the amino acids, much less fat storage, and less stress on your liver and kidneys to digest, filter, and excrete the byproducts.

Is all protein the same? Yes and no. Remember, the body doesn't really know whether you're eating an egg, a slice of roast beef, or a plate of beans and rice. All it understands and responds to is using the maximum number of amino acids in the correct proportions. So although the egg is the most "complete" protein in that it contains all the amino acids, and the roast beef is nearly as complete, the body isn't going to use all that protein. There's very little storage capacity for amino acids—just a bit in the liver—so after the requisite amino acids have been used for tissue repair, the rest are converted to fat and the excess nitrogen produced will be excreted.

You may need a little animal protein in your diet, but not nearly as much as most Americans eat. Complex carbohydrates contribute significant amounts of useable protein to your diet with more fiber, less fat, and far less waste than animal protein. Many vegetables contain incomplete proteins, that is, they don't have enough of the essential eight amino acids to sustain growth. But when you eat vegetables in combination, they give you exactly what you need—no more, no less. You don't have to eat them at the same meal; they can be eaten later that day and they'll still combine perfectly well to form complete proteins.

Some traditional, delicious mixes of vegetable protein are:

- rice and beans
- corn tortillas and beans
- bulgur wheat and chick-peas
- barley and a stew of carrots, turnips, and greens
- pasta in a tomato-mushroom sauce

Eating less animal protein and more complex carbohydrates is like running your car on unleaded fuel. The body, like the automobile, will run more efficiently, get more miles to the gallon (the ability to feel good all day long), and will even run faster (with more energy and less fatigue).

Who Really Needs Excess Protein?

Some of us certainly do need more protein than the rest of us. Children through adolescence, pregnant and lactating women, burn victims, and people who've been malnourished for months do need additional protein—as much as 120 grams a day. When proteins are synthesized and broken down in children, they are used to enhance growth. In a pregnant or nursing woman, the amino acids are building tissue for another human being. In a severely ill or injured person, the amino acids are replenishing the damaged tissue.[2]

And though a newborn baby and a child need large amounts of dietary protein relative to their body weight while they're growing, adults and elderly people need very little—only one gram of protein for every three pounds of body weight daily.

The Documented Evidence: Laboratory Findings on Protein

I began looking into the amazing effect that too much protein had on every system of the body. Many researchers—biochemists, molecular biologists, nutritionists, and gerontologists—had supplied me with copious documentation from recent studies on laboratory animals and humans indicating that low-protein eating was the way to go.

Dr. Vernon R. Young and Dr. Peter L. Pellett in the Department of Applied Biological Sciences at M.I.T. did metabolic balance studies on rats and humans. They found that "high-protein diets may cause a deterioration in body calcium balance. The major effect of a high-protein diet appears to be located at the level of the kidney, and the mechanism is associated with a reduced reabsorption of filtered calcium . . . high-protein diets may contribute to the etiology of osteoporosis in the adult population."[3]

Drs. Barry M. Brenner, Timothy W. Meyer, and Thomas H. Hostetter from the Laboratory of Kidney and Electrolyte Physiology and the Department of Medicine, Brigham and Women's Hospital, and Harvard Medical School studied a reduction of kidney function in rats on high-protein diets. They found that rats could live much longer even after the removal of five-sixths of their kidneys if they were fed a low-protein diet.[4]

One of the best-known researchers in the longevity field, Dr. Roy L. Walford, currently participating in the Biosphere II experiment in Arizona, cites undernutrition as one of the main factors in increasing life span in many species. He wrote in the April 1990 issue of *Geriatrics*, "Although DR [dietary restriction] affects a wide spectrum of biological processes, the two aspects of DR that are clinically relevant are its ability to maintain the vitality of the immune system and to reduce the incidence of age-related diseases. While these effects alone do not necessarily promote longevity, a strong immune system and a reduced disease incidence have tremendous impact on a patient's latter-year productivity and quality of life." He goes on to explain undernutrition, or restriction of calories in the diet, and concludes that "it has been observed that animals on a protein-deficient diet tend to eat less and thus voluntarily restrict their caloric intake."[5]

How Protein Affects Your
Internal Organs

Let me give you a rundown on each of the body's organs and processes and how protein affects their potential.

THE KIDNEY

The kidney is the body's filter. Nearly a quarter of the blood your heart pumps every minute must go through the kidneys, which spins off urea, a waste product produced when the cells burn energy. Urea is removed from the blood as urine through the kidneys.

Your kidneys shrink as you get older, and they lose a certain percentage of their function each year. By the time you're 50, you've lost about 15 percent of this function, and by the time you're 80, you may have lost 30 to 40 percent. Certain kidney cells do regenerate but others do not. You can manage with the number you have left well into old age if the demands on the kidney aren't too great. But a high-protein diet puts an unfair load on them. They have to work much harder to handle all the water that extra protein's excess nitrogen requires in processing and, consequently, excrete more minerals along with the water and urea.

As the kidneys work harder and more kidney cells are destroyed that can't be replaced, the fewer remaining cells have more trouble filtering out the toxins your body must get rid of. These toxins back up in the bloodstream. Kidney dysfunction can also cause high blood pressure; and high blood pressure puts even more stress on the kidneys, causing them to degenerate rapidly.

There's no way for a kidney to regain the function it's lost. When the kidneys stop working, so does your body. Unlike a heart, which can be patched and mended and bypassed, there is no way to "fix" a damaged kidney. Dialysis, a process whereby the blood is "cleansed" in a machine and then returned to your body, is a painful and not always successful procedure. Kidney disease is a silent and deadly killer.

You can, however, keep your kidneys in peak condition by being absolutely sure that they don't have to do any more work than they should. The kidneys are the most vital organs in your body in terms of the aging process. They can maintain that all-important nitrogen balance for years at full functioning capacity, depending on the fuel you give them to process. As you now know, the less protein they have to deal with, the more efficiently they'll work.

For years, nephrologists have been using an extremely low protein diet in conjunction with dialysis for their patients with great success. As a matter of fact, a reputed renal nutritionist in Boulder, Colorado, Barbara Kantor, has found that by simply putting her patients with minimal kidney dysfunction on a low-protein diet, she can reverse their prognosis and spare them from dialysis. A low-protein diet alone can lower the BUN or blood/urea/nitrogen count from a high of 40 to a normal 20 in just one month.

Excess protein causes dehydration. During the blood-filtering process, the kidneys must excrete a great deal of water to get rid of excess nitrogen. (The body must be in nitrogen balance, but eating protein gives us more nitrogen than we can use.) Excreting so much water impairs athletic performance by robbing the muscles of the water they need so badly when they're under stress.

Dr. Barry Brenner at Brigham and Women's Hospital in Boston has extensively studied the effects of dietary composition on renal function.[6] He cites some studies done on dogs in the 1950s by Addis[7] that showed that eating a lot of protein was causing such a burden on the kidneys that they had to be in use more or less continuously. They never got a chance to rest. All that energy going just to move waste out of the body!

A human study on sixty-four patients over eighteen months conducted by Dr. Benno Ihle from the Department of Nephrology of the Royal Melbourne Hospital in Victoria, Australia, reported that patients with renal disease on very low protein diets (0.18 grams protein per pound of body weight per day) drastically improved their chances. End-stage renal failure developed in 27 percent of those on a regular diet, but in only 6 percent of the group on the low-protein diet.[8]

The first national study of renal disease ever mandated by Congress—the MDRD study—began in 1984 and is currently underway at fifteen medical centers across the country. Dr. John Kusek of the National Institutes of Health, director of the study, hopes to prove that a low-protein diet is the best therapy for kidney patients. The patients are being maintained on three different amounts of protein consumption, and results will probably start coming in next year.[9]

THE BONES

Protein also robs the bones of the calcium they so desperately need. In 1920, the first studies were done indicating that excess protein intake caused an increase in urinary calcium excretion. I have already cited the famous Eskimo study[10] that proved that the acidic effect of a meat diet causes calcium loss, which in turn causes the bones to become fragile.

One interesting British study compared the bone density of twenty-five vegetarians to twenty-five omnivores. The subjects, who ranged in age from 50 to 79, showed a marked difference in bone density—those who consumed no animal protein had startlingly denser bones than their protein-eating colleagues.[11]

In addition, excess animal protein causes kidney stones; a high-protein diet has an adverse effect on the chemical composition of urine and allows calcium deposits to form in the kidneys.[12]

THE LIVER

All the toxins and waste that result from the chemical reactions of your body must be processed by the liver and then excreted by the kidney. If you eat too much protein, these two vital organs have a great deal of extra work to do and can become overtaxed.

The liver's function is to help purify the body. The largest and most metabolically complex organ in the body, it formulates and excretes bile, regulates carbohydrate balance, synthesizes fats, controls cholesterol metabolism, forms urea (a waste byproduct spun off by the red blood cells), and other proteins, and metabolizes and detoxifies foreign substances in the body, such as alcohol or drugs.

Excess protein is metabolized and stored by the liver, and it's common to see elevated counts of liver enzymes (SGOT, SGPT) and other liver function tests (alkaline phosphatase, bilirubin, and total protein) in patients consuming high-protein diets. These values, however, can return to normal or below normal within six months on a low-protein diet.

Most of the breakdown of amino acids takes place in the liver. This organ actually processes everything you eat and metabolizes the useful elements for cell maintenance and repair. But when the liver is overtaxed and starts to lose its function, there is very little warning. When it's no longer working properly, the body can't sustain itself. Although the liver has wonderful regenerative properties, it can be destroyed by excess consumption of alcohol. And it can be badly stressed by excess consumption of protein.[13] According to Dr. T. Colin Campbell, protein increases the enzyme activity that converts the chemicals in the foods we consume and in the environment around us to carcinogens, and protein promotes the binding of these carcinogens to DNA. When he tried to induce tumors in rats, he found that the enzyme activity required to produce a carcinogen from aflatoxins (molds typically used to grow cancers) was greatly reduced on a low-protein diet.[14]

Dr. Linda Youngman, one of the researchers in Dr. Campbell's Chinese study who has recently moved to the University of California at Berkeley, performed a two-and-a-half-year tumor study on eight hundred Fisher-344 rats on either 6-, 14-, or 22-percent protein diets. Those fed the lowest amount of protein had far fewer tumors, both chemically induced and spontaneous, and a lower incidence of metastases, i.e., the cancers didn't spread.

She tried shifting some high-protein-diet rats with existing tumors to a low-protein diet. This switch prevented further growth of the tumors in almost all cases. But when she shifted low-protein eaters to a high-protein diet, the tumors took off.[15]

THE COLON

My next thought was to look at the way high-protein diets affected the colon. Many studies I read indicated that high intake of red meat had a strong correlation with an increased incidence of colon cancer. The rate of colon cancer in Far Eastern and developing nations, where there just isn't much animal protein available, was staggeringly lower than in America.

Dr. Walter C. Willett from the Harvard Medical School and

Brigham and Women's Hospital made some very interesting findings over a ten-year period. He studied over 88,000 women ages 34 to 59 and found that the relative risk of colon cancer in those who consumed beef, pork, or lamb as a main dish every day was nearly two and a half times higher than those who ate meat less than once a month.[16] Because animal protein is digested much more slowly than plant protein, any carcinogens or toxic agents present in the animal protein will be in contact with your digestive organs for much longer—so the cancer rates make sense.

BLOOD-SUGAR LEVELS

High-protein diets slow the absorption of glucose from the bloodstream to the cells, the result being elevated blood-sugar levels. And as we age, blood sugar increases. In diabetes, for example, we find that there is an autoimmune reaction in the islets of Langerhans in the pancreas so they overreact and can't produce insulin, which transports glucose from the bloodstream to the cells of the body, thus lowering blood sugar. A low-protein diet has been found to facilitate glucose absorption to the cells. And since diabetics are seventeen times more prone to renal failure than other individuals, it is crucial to reduce the protein in their diet in order to protect their kidney function.

A low-protein diet has also reduced the risk of pancreatic cancer. A study by noted researchers Farrow and Davis showed that risk of pancreatic cancer increased as protein intake increased, although not as fat intake increased.[17]

THE HEART

It almost seems redundant by now to talk about preserving the cardiovascular system with low-protein eating, but I do want to mention a two-year test in France. The researchers showed that rats on a 50-percent protein diet had more vascular aging—as shown in thickened and less elastic aortas—than the rats on a 10-percent protein diet. A higher-protein diet resulted in a deterioration of muscle fibers of the heart, thus causing cardiac function to fail and precipitating congestive heart failure.[18]

Heart function and coronary artery blood flow improve dramatically when the patient is placed on a low-protein diet. In fact, Dr. Dean Ornish's life-style heart trial, a study performed at the University of California, San Francisco, School of Medicine, showed a reversal of blocked coronary arteries on such a diet.[19]

The Low-Protein Breakthrough in My Medical Practice

I had, of course, kept my kidney patients on a low-protein diet for years. But I still hesitated about introducing the low-protein concept to patients who had no kidney trouble. The traditional thinking was that patients who need to lose weight or control blood pressure would do fine if they just reduced the fat and sugar in their diets. I wasn't enough of a maverick to start a revolution against respected physicians who'd never even considered protein as an issue in weight loss or longevity.

And yet I saw that many of my patients were having trouble losing weight or lowering blood pressure on the standard low-fat, low-calorie diets. They'd do fine for a while, then stop complying and fall right back into old patterns. Their weight and blood pressure would zoom back up; they'd feel depressed and punish themselves with a lot of guilt and anxiety.

It was then that I knew I had to implement the low-protein diet for all my patients. I felt completely confident from the reading I'd done and from my own experience that it was time to start spreading the news. If nothing else, the diet would do for my patients what it had done for me—given me boundless energy, a positive outlook on life, and the will to go further than I ever had before. I figured that if I could succeed in giving my patients an infusion of that great low-protein feeding, they'd gain the stamina and self-esteem to stick with their diets.

The low-protein program became the foundation of all my patients' "wellness routines," as I decided to call them. I implemented the diet at the Southwest Health Institute, which I founded in Phoenix in 1980 and which is dedicated to applying preventive medicine to improve the quality and possibly the quantity of life.

I'd been hopeful about the results for at least a few of my patients, but what actually happened surpassed my greatest expectations.

Those who had never before been able to lose weight and keep it off were shocked to find that they were eating more and losing more at the same time. Their blood and kidney profiles improved, their desire and ability to start an exercise program and keep it up skyrocketed. They began to reduce their medications as their disease syndromes lessened. Patients with diabetes, kidney disease, arthritis, early osteoporosis, high blood pressure, and chronic obesity all improved.

Fifteen years after I began my own personal low-protein diet, I realized that, in effect, I had slowed down my own aging process. Today, at age 47, my blood tests, including liver function, kidney function, cholesterol, trigylcerides, and oxygen uptake are all the same as when I first started my personal low-protein program fifteen years ago. I feel better and younger now than I did then.

Let me add that whenever anyone tries to guess my age, they invariably peg me as 34 or 35. I think it's important to let you know that once you start on this breakthrough nutritional program, no one will ever know how old you really are.

Don't tell—why should you? I haven't until now.

How Much Protein Is Just Enough?

Nutritionists have gone back and forth for years on how much dietary protein adults actually need. The National Research Council's current recommended daily amount, or RDA, is .8 grams per kilogram of body weight (or about 1 gram for every 3 pounds that you weigh). Following this recommendation, along with other published dietary guidelines, should put your protein intake at about 12 to 15 percent of daily calories. However, most people are consuming three to four times the council's recommendation, as well as ignoring other dietary guidelines, the result being a dangerously high percentage of their daily calories coming from protein and fat. What's worse, about 70 percent of that already high protein intake is coming from animal foods.

I'm sticking with the council's recommendations—to a point—and I will be telling you how to achieve them. I feel you can be perfectly healthy if about 15 percent of your daily calories comes from protein, as long as *most of it comes from plant rather than animal sources.* Let me emphasize that I am not excluding animal foods, only limiting them, and you'll be allowed ample flexibility in food choices. Remember, the Anti-Aging Diet is intended as a long-life plan, and, as such, it's got to be enjoyable and practical for you over the many decades to come.

Now, let me summarize the benefits of a low-protein diet:

- slower aging
- lower dietary fat and cholesterol intake
- decreased strain on the liver and kidneys
- stronger immune system
- decreased nitrogen intake
- decreased loss of body minerals (particularly calcium) through excretion
- increased amounts of complex carbohydrates and therefore
- increased amounts of fiber, vitamin E, and beta carotene
- increased amount of food possible on a diet and therefore
- decrease in hunger
- better weight control
- lower LDL cholesterol levels; i.e., lower total cholesterol
- lower risk of heart disease
- lower risk of cancer

This book is the practical application of my anti-aging diet—the perfect way for you to incorporate low-protein eating into your personal life-style for greater health and longevity.

Chapter 4

Less Protein, More Health

My patients at the Southwest Health Institute are the very best proof I can offer that the Anti-Aging Diet works. Some have been with me for the past fifteen years—seeing me for "wellness" check-ups once a year—and others have come more recently, to lose weight, to make life-style changes and, hopefully, to live better today and for many more tomorrows.

I want to share with you now some of my most remarkable cases. My anti-aging diet, this revolutionary way of eating, has changed my patients' lives—in many cases, actually saved lives. Simply by reducing dietary protein, my patients have, within six months:

- lost the desired amount of weight and kept it off
- reversed kidney disease
- restored liver functions to normal
- controlled hypertension
- lowered cholesterol and triglyceride levels
- relieved arthritis
- controlled diabetes
- stopped the progression of osteoporosis
- prevented a progression of, or reversed, coronary artery disease thus obviating the need for surgical intervention

I have also seen remission of certain cancers in some of my patients. Although low-protein eating has undoubtedly made a difference in strengthening their immune systems and removing toxins from their bodies, it must be pointed out that diet alone cannot control cancer. It can, however, become a vital part of any treatment program involving surgery and/or chemotherapy by allowing a patient to become stronger so that he or she can tolerate any medical treatment program that might be implemented.

How I Introduced the Anti-Aging Diet to My Patients

I initially proposed the Anti-Aging Diet to my kidney patients and called it the "semi-vegetarian diet." It reduced protein intake to 15 percent of total daily caloric consumption, and this protein was to be vegetable protein with a small amount of chicken and fish. I told my patients that a 15-percent protein diet such as the one I had developed would get their kidney function tests back into the normal range. I was, of course, curious to see whether their incidence of heart disease, diabetes, gastrointestinal problems, and elevated cholesterol levels would be lower than those of my patients on a standard protein diet. Over time, I was amazed to see the divergence of the two groups. After five years, those on the low-protein diet had a 50 percent lower incidence of all those conditions.

In one of my most successful cases, a woman named Christina came to me at age 31, looking and feeling as though she were 50. Christina was 40 pounds overweight when she first came to see me. She was taking five different medications to control heart palpitations, depression and anxiety, elevated cholesterol, and headaches. She'd been taking all these drugs for the past five years and also trying to lose weight with every fad diet that came along.

Thirty days after I put Christina on the Anti-Aging Diet, she had lost 25 pounds and I'd weaned her off every medication except the one for her headaches. Sixty days later, she had lost 40 pounds and didn't need even an aspirin to feel wonderful. Her blood pressure had gone down from 150/90 to 120/80; her cholesterol had been reduced from 260 to 180; her triglycerides had dropped dramatically from 220 to 100. It's now three years since I met Christina—she never gained a pound back, is walking several miles a day, and confidently tells me she'll be leading a low-protein lifestyle from now on.

Then there's Ted. He visited my office several years ago when he was 46. He'd been seen by a leading cardiovascular surgeon who recommended a bypass for his blocked coronary artery. Ted was nervous about his chances, but more than a little terrified of the proposed $20,000 surgery.

In less than three months on the Anti-Aging Diet, he was off all medication, walking six miles daily, and in fabulously good health. The last time I saw Ted, he'd lost 30 pounds and his EKG indicated that his heart was in perfect shape.

Another exemplary patient is Evangeline, 44 years old, a member of the National Speakers' Association, and a wonderful communications manager. When she first came to see me, she weighed 350 pounds. Her blood pressure was 180/110, her triglycerides were 200, and she never exercised because she was too exhausted to walk even a mile a day.

In one year, she was down to 220 pounds, her blood pressure was 130/80; her triglycerides were 70. She hasn't yet obtained her ideal weight, but she's very encouraged about her improvement and tells me the diet really made it easy for her. She walks four miles a day and has an incredible energy level. She told me recently, "I thought that I would weigh over 300 pounds until the day I died. This weight loss has changed my life. I will never, ever be heavy again."

Another interesting patient of mine is a former "proteinaholic" named John, 57 years old, a driven salesman who was inexorable in the pursuit of the deal. His kidneys were failing and his liver tests were elevated from years of chronic alcohol consumption. Typically, he ate beef three times a day.

I told him that if he wanted to live, he was going to have to make radical changes in his life-style—get off the booze and meat entirely. Few patients were as difficult to convince of the potential benefits of the Anti-Aging Diet as John. However, few have enjoyed a success as remarkable as his. Within six months, his kidney tests were absolutely normal and his liver function tests were almost within normal range. He had energy for the first time in three years. And today, twelve years later, John is still sober and still eating a low-protein diet.

Then there's Delia. She's 39 years old and works as a Social Security administrator. When she first came to see me, she was severely diabetic. Her blood sugar was over 400 (a normal level is 70 to 120 milligrams per deciliter) and she weighed 340 pounds—which at five feet, five inches tall was an incredible load for her frame. Her blood pressure was 160/100, and she was taking medication for high blood pressure when I met her. Genetically, she hadn't been dealt any good cards, either. Her father had died at the age of 49 of a heart attack; her siblings were all overweight. She was so depressed when she walked into my office, I could hardly convince her that she was about to undergo some major improvements in her health on the Anti-Aging Diet.

We've known for years that diet has a great impact on diabetes. Initially, researchers felt that sugar was the major culprit in this disease; then obesity was found to be a decisive factor, as well; and, of course, the amount of fat in the diet plays a part.

But it is increasingly evident that many of the complications of adult-onset diabetes, including kidney failure, are greatly influenced by the amount of protein in the diet.

The mechanism of diabetes is an autoimmune reaction in which the islets of Langerhans in the pancreas can't produce insulin. It is insulin that transports glucose into the cells, thus lowering the level of sugar in the blood. Without insulin, the blood sugar level rises too high. I've found that a low-protein diet makes an enormous difference for my diabetic patients because it facilitates glucose absorption from the bloodstream to the various cells of the body. The more fiber and complex carbohydrate the body has to work with, the easier the absorption of glucose is into the cells, and eating less protein means you can more easily eat more carbohydrates.

Within a year of starting the program, Delia had lost 150 pounds and her blood pressure was much more nearly normal—120/80. But what was more astounding was that her blood sugar was completely normal at 110 milligrams. When I told her she no longer had diabetes, she started to cry. With tears streaming from her eyes, she thanked me for helping her to regain her life.

Tex was referred to me after a severe bout of angina had sent him to the emergency room in an ambulance. At 55, he had astronomically high blood pressure and blocked coronary arteries, and he never exercised. He couldn't see the benefits of the diet I outlined and was adamant about it. "I'm a cowboy and was raised on meat and eggs. There's no way that I'm gonna give up beef for being healthy," said Tex. But he changed his mind when I told him quietly that I didn't think he had a chance of surviving a massive heart attack. Several months later Tex was beef free, ran three miles a day, and had no chest pain. He confessed to me, when he came to see me for a routine checkup, that he'd grown to love spinach and brown rice casseroles—as long as they were spiced up with lots of salsa.

I also want to tell you about a patient of mine who's a well-known rock star—let's call him Mark, though that's not his real name. When I met him, he was 45 and addicted to a variety of substances, including alcohol and barbiturates, which he took to get himself to sleep but which, in fact, made his insomnia worse. His career was on the downslide and he had the good sense to realize that getting his health back had a lot to do with his creative potential. He got on the Anti-Aging Diet, started bicycling six miles a day, and came to see me frequently for pep talks on the long-term benefits of what this new life-style had to offer. Within three months, he was no longer drinking alcohol and was completely off the sleeping medication, his insomnia had been resolved, and his career was taking a great turn for the better.

Look at the incredible physiological and biochemical changes that took place: When he came to see me, his cholesterol was 330, but in three months it was down to 190. His blood pressure decreased from 160/100 to 120/80, and his weight went from 210 to 170. Because of his heavy drinking, his liver function tests initially indicated 8 scores elevated out of 10, but in three months he was down to normal on all but one of those. And his kidney function dropped from a high of 25 to a normal 17 during this period.

Another of my patients, whom we'll call Lois, is the daughter of

RESULTS OF TWENTY TYPICAL PATIENTS ON THE ANTI-AGING-DIET

	Age	Weight		Blood Pressure		Cholesterol		Triglycerides		BUN		Comments
		Initial	Improved	Initial	Improved	Initial	Improved	Initial	Improved	Initial	Improved	
Debbie	27	200	135	normal		normal		normal		—		Lowest weight since age 16, achieved in 4 months
Christina	31	180	140	150/90	120/80	260	180	220	100	—		Off five medications; weight stabilized over 3 years on the diet
Denise	36	200	140	160/90	120/80	270	160					Weight stabilized; hypertension reversed
Betty	38	191	120	140/90	110/70	280	200			—		Weight and cholesterol reduced in 15 months
Delia	39	340	190	160/100	120/80	220	160					Glucose from 405 to 110; diabetes cured
Jennifer	30	340	140	180/100	110/70	400	150			22	15	Lost two hundred pounds over 2 years
Helena	35	160	115	130/80	110/70	220	140	—		19	12	Off antidepressants in 3 months
Alice	36	210	120	130/80	110/70	260	145	—		—		Lost 90 pounds in 9 months
Mark	45	210	170	160/100	120/80	330	190			25	17	In 3 months was off drugs and alcohol
Peter	34	180	160	140/90	130/80	295	180			24	19	"Addicted" to health in 3 months

John	48	195 175	150/90 on medication 120/80 without medication	380 175	—	30 18	Improvement in 6 months
Guy	53	215 165	140/90 120/80	290 180	—	20 16	Off all medication; impotence no longer evident
Evangeline	44	350 200	180/110 130/80	290 190	200 70	—	Improvement in 1 year
Norman	48	215 180	160/100 120/80	—	—	—	In 6 months reversed liver disease
Helen	73	146 120	120/80 on medication 122/84 without medication	248 220	172 100	21 16	Off all medication in 7 months
Adele	84	180 140	140/80 110/70	258 220	354 210	32 17	Reversed kidney disease
Don	85	175 175	180/100 140/70	285 185	230 100	—	Controlled hypertension and cholesterol; off all medication
Florence	86	141 138	170/100 130/90	normal	normal	36 16	Reversed kidney disease
Reuben	90	155 141	180/120 130/80	254 210	171 106	—	Lowered blood pressure in 3 months; off all medication
Lucy	91	116 116	normal	normal	normal	39 18	Reversed kidney disease

a U.S. senator. She is 19 years old, beautiful, bright, articulate, charming, and bulimic. In a desperate attempt to please her father, she started purging food at the age of 12 in order to lose weight and turn herself into some impossible approximation of her image of ideal beauty.

For years she had been forcing all her feelings beneath the surface, but by the time she came to see me she had really begun to fear for her life. It took us six months to make the breakthrough and control her bulimia. She said that the Anti-Aging Diet had helped to steady her emotionally as well as physically. She just wasn't afraid to eat and gain weight because she felt so good from the nutritious food and daily exercise that she was more able to work with her feelings and bring them out. She stopped purging and maintained a normal weight of 122.

I don't include the rest of her clinical statistics because, to me, the most important result in her case was the apparent emotional growth that allowed her to escape from a self-imposed prison.

And for those doubters who will say that radical change can only happen in a fairly young body, let me tell you about Lucy Brown, who just celebrated her ninety-first birthday. She's been my patient for almost twenty years and probably knows as much about low-protein eating as I do. When I first examined Lucy, she was dying of renal failure, which was undoubtedly more serious than her blocked coronary arteries and her high cholesterol count. Her kidney function tests really worried me—her BUN score was 39 (about 20 is normal), and her creatinine was 2.1 (normal is under 1.3). After six months on the diet, Lucy's scores were all in the normal range and her other blood tests were as good as those of a healthy 20-year-old.

Low-Protein Data from China

There's just one more body of evidence I must tell you about. I mention it because it's a huge survey conducted over many years, and it corroborates all of my evidence from the 10,000 patients I've seen at the Southwest Health Institute. This study, currently still underway in China, has in fact changed the nature of human participation in dietary studies, and the sheer numbers of participants will convince you—as it did me—that the low-protein lifestyle is the healthiest course you can adopt.

You've probably noticed that most of the interesting scientific data on protein has come out of laboratory experiments with rats, guinea pigs, hamsters, and the like. The reason for this is that it's practically impossible to get a control group of human beings to comply with any diet for a period of years without deviating from the required nutritional model. In China, however, where people have eaten basically the same diet for thousands of years, and where a government-sponsored plan guarantees compliance, it was possible to get 6,500 individuals to participate in a nine-year epidemiological study.

The Chinese data comes from a joint study engineered by scientists from Cornell University, Oxford University, and the Chinese Academy of Preventive Medicine in Beijing. The National Cancer Institute and the Chinese government provide the major funding for this extraordinary survey with additional support from the American Institute for Cancer Research, the United States Food and Drug Administration, the United Kingdom Imperial Cancer Research Fund, and some private American companies.

Dr. T. Colin Campbell, a nutritional biochemist from Cornell University, is the American director of this study, which will be going on for the next forty to fifty years. He was initially excited about conducting his research in China because he had in this "living laboratory" a vast number of people all over a huge country who had been consuming basically the same, unvaried, low-protein diet all their lives and were happy to answer questions about their eating habits.[1]

Who Eats What?

It's difficult to separate protein from fat in most human studies, because most humans are omnivores and consume animal rather than vegetable protein. When you eat meat, you get fat along with your protein. But the Chinese eat virtually no dairy products and meat is served as a condiment or flavoring in dishes rather than as a main course. The largest percentage of protein intake in America comes from animal products: in the United States, 70 percent of total daily calories are from protein; in China it is only 7 percent.[2]

Americans consume approximately 10 to 12 grams of dietary fiber per day; the Chinese mean intake is a whopping 34 to 77 daily grams. The fat in the Chinese diet is exceptionally low, too. Just 15 percent of the total calories in the typical Chinese diet come from fat; most Americans have a fat intake of about 40 percent of total calories. Interestingly enough, though the Chinese only consume a little over 500 milligrams of calcium a day, as compared with the American average of 1,150 milligrams, there is little or no osteoporosis in China. You will remember, of course, that we lose calcium rapidly when we consume lots of protein.

And finally, the big news on calories. The Chinese intake is on average 2,600 calories a day—which is much more than most Americans eat. Even so, obesity is rarely if ever a problem in China. My point is—what makes you fat is not the calories; it's the protein. It becomes even more evident when you look at the Chinese study that calorie consumption has very little to do with weight loss or maintenance. As you reduce your protein, you'll be able to eat more calories a day and not gain weight!

This phenomenon has also been demonstrated in Dr. Campbell's laboratory at Cornell University. Drs. Ronda Bell and Linda Youngman did a study showing that rats fed a low-protein diet expend more energy per gram of food intake than animals on a high-protein diet, even though the low-protein group is consuming more calories. The researchers kept their animals at five different protein levels: 4, 8, 12, 16, and 20 percent of total calories. The groups fed the lowest amount of protein ate more, weighed less, and developed far fewer tumors than the groups fed high protein. The low-protein-diet rats were alert and energetic and exercised voluntarily far more than the high-protein-diet groups—one rat typically ran nine miles a day, another would grab onto his activity wheel and spin wildly for hours![3]

Diseases of Affluence versus Diseases of Poverty

Some of Dr. Campbell's most interesting findings show up when we compare disease patterns in America and China.[4] You'll notice that there are really two types of mortal illness: diseases of poverty, which are found primarily in underdeveloped countries that lack adequate sanitation and immunization; and diseases of affluence, which result basically from abuse of the extraordinary abundance more developed nations enjoy. Americans typically suffer from cardiovascular disease, kidney disease, obesity, diabetes, and cancers of the stomach, liver, colon, breast, and lung.

CUMULATIVE MORTALITY RATES PER 100,000 PEOPLE IN CHINA AND THE U.S. (AGES FROM BIRTH TO 64)

	CHINA Male	Female	U.S. Male	Female
Colon cancer	2.4	1.6	5.8	4.4
Lung cancer	8.0	3.5	26.9	12.5
Coronary artery disease	4.0	3.4	66.8	18.9
Breast cancer	——	3.1	——	15.1

It is also useful to compare plasma cholesterol levels in the two countries. In China, the average range is between 85 to 170; in America, it's rare to find an adult with a cholesterol level under 180!

And for those who claim that the basic American problem with cholesterol and diet in general is just too much fat, let me counter with Dr. Campbell's statement: "I would like to advance the hypothesis that the much higher mortality rates for so-called diseases of affluence in the United States are accounted for by the much greater consumption of animal products and it is not just the higher levels of saturated fat in these products that account for this effect. . . . And, of course, the flip side of this hypothesis must recognize that as animal food intake goes up, plant food consumption goes down. When, in turn, the nutritional properties of plant foods are examined, the preponderance of evidence suggests a large variety of protective constituents."[5]

Dr. Campbell and his colleagues didn't tell me anything my patients and I didn't already know—a low-protein life-style is the best preventive medicine around.

Yes, there is life after animal product consumption—a life that will make you stronger, healthier, and less susceptible to life-threatening diseases. Turn the page and you'll find out how to implement the anti-aging diet for yourself.

Part Two

The Anti-Aging
Life-style

Chapter 5

The Anti-Aging Diet

The Anti-Aging Diet is unlike any diet you've ever tried to follow. It's easy; as simple as $2 + 2 = 4$.

You are allowed one animal protein food per day—no more, no less.

That's the only rule you have to remember. And once you've determined how many *grams* of protein you should be eating each day (see How Many Grams Are Right for You, pages 71–72), you'll wonder why the concept of calorie- or fat-counting was ever invented. Unlike tasteless, complex weight-reduction diets that require ingredients from all ends of the earth and a brilliant mathematician to figure proportions and quantities, this diet is sublimely delicious and easy to follow.

For example, you may eat:

- two eggs for breakfast *or*
- a chicken sandwich for lunch *or*
- one fillet of fish for dinner

And that's it. That's all the animal protein you need to stay healthy *and* lose weight. The rest of your protein will come from vegetable sources, legumes, and grains—the other food groups that have somehow gotten lost in the shuffle and on the back shelves of your cupboard.

Forget About Calories!

In the Anti-Aging Diet, there is *no* calorie counting. There's no starving yourself, either! You will find that in two easy, comfortable stages you'll change your perspective on what a well-balanced, delicious meal consists of. You'll know exactly how to shop, cook, and put meals together creatively. By making up your total daily calorie intake of **20 percent protein, 20 percent fats, and 60 percent complex carbohydrates**, you will naturally and simply lose weight, keep it off, feel wonderful, and extend your life span.

A Diet That Makes You Feel Wonderful

Most Americans consume about 120 grams of protein a day. My Anti-Aging Diet calls for about half that. But what you lose in protein, you more than make up for in the quantity and quality of food you'll be eating. You will not feel weak, you will not feel starved or jealous of high-protein eaters around you. You will, in fact, feel so good while you're on this diet that you will begin to wonder why you never ate this way before. It's not a three-week or three-month plan that leaves your body thinner and your emotions frayed and ragged as you find yourself craving forbidden foods and feeling deprived and frustrated. It is not so much a diet as a long-term gift you can give yourself.

You probably hate dieting—everybody does—because it keeps you away from all the things you love. You punish yourself by restricting your food intake and, in fact, you do lose weight. But at what cost!

The problem with a "punishing" diet is that it makes you alter your natural eating patterns for the duration of the diet—usually about the time it takes you to get through your new diet book. As soon as you reach your ideal weight and go back to eating the way you used to, you regain the weight. It's a sad fact that 90 percent of all dieters gain back every ounce they've lost within two years of their diet.

I promise that this will *not* happen when you're on my groundbreaking low-protein diet. While you're following the Anti-Aging Diet, you'll be losing weight gradually—perhaps at the rate of two pounds a week—but very consistently. When you are within five pounds of your goal weight, you'll switch to the lifetime program and add on portions (and therefore calories) that will help you maintain your weight. You will find that for the first time in your life you'll be able to keep weight off effortlessly and tone up every system in your body by making low-protein eating the foundation of your anti-aging program.

Why the Anti-Aging Diet Works

Everybody's diet is made up of three elements: carbohydrate, fat, and protein. Carbohydrate is the preferred fuel for your body because it metabolizes so efficiently. When you consume a diet high in complex carbohydrates—salads, fruits, grains, cereals, and vegetables—as opposed to refined carbohydrates like sugar, you will be supplying your body with a high-fiber, low-protein, low-fat diet which will be naturally low in calories.

After your body processes the complex carbohydrates you eat, the next element it processes is fat. But if you aren't very active, your body stores those fats away for some future time when they may be needed for excess energy. Where do those fat stores end up? You've probably guessed it already—they end up as unwanted, ugly pounds.

The last element your body processes is protein. It takes your body almost a day to digest and excrete a steak, which means a great deal of stress and a lot of extra work for the liver and kidney.

By lowering your intake of protein and fat—each to 20 percent of your total daily calories—while you're losing weight, you'll feel an immediate boost of energy. You won't feel hungry because you can consume more complex carbohydrates than protein or fat for the same number of calories. One hundred grams of meat equal 200 calories; whereas 500 grams of complex carbohydrates give you the same 200 calories.

There are no *forbidden* foods on this diet. I do want you to keep the amount of caffeine and alcohol you consume to an absolute minimum, particularly while you are losing weight. Caffeine stimulates your central nervous system, causing you to experience mood swings. Alcohol is a depressant and has a negative effect on your immune system. Also, it has no nutritive value, only empty calories, and it tends to make you less conscientious about sticking to your new food plan.

But everything else you're accustomed to eating is permitted on the Anti-Aging Diet—in reasonable amounts. You can even have snacks—there are several great ones suggested on the individual menu plans. I think you'll find, however, that protein-rich foods just won't taste as good to you as they used to. And, after a few months, you may discover you don't even want animal protein every day. You may at that point choose to limit your intake to four or five times a week.

How to Count Grams of Protein

Generations of diet books have taught us all about calories—a calorie is a measurement of how much energy the food you eat contains. It's a very vague concept, actually, unlike the absolute of a gram, which is very concrete.

A gram is a measurement of weight—it shows you how big something is. It takes about 28 grams to make an ounce. Most individuals eat between 300 and 400 grams of food per day. You don't really need to be concerned with the weight of what you're eating, though. All you have to know is that only 20 percent of your daily calories will come from protein while you're losing weight, and the most protein is found in animal products. So if you become familiar with the following continuum of weights, you'll be able to gauge your allotment for each meal pretty well:

PROTEIN CONTENT OF POPULAR FOODS

	Serving Size	Grams of Protein
Fruit, any uncooked	3½ ounces	0
Coffee, tea, water, soda	8 ounces	0
Vegetables, green	½ cup	2
Potato, plain baked	4 ounces or medium	2
Rice, plain cooked	½ cup	2
Bagel, roll, bread	1, 1 slice	2
Egg white	1	3
Cereal, ready to eat	½ cup	3
Pasta, plain, cooked	1 cup	4
Egg, whole	1	6
Cheese, Cheddar	1 ounce	7
Sunflower seeds	1 ounce	7
Beans, lentils, cooked	½ cup	8 to 10
Skim milk	1 cup	8
Shrimp	3 ounces	21
Meat, 85% lean burger	3 ounces	22
Poultry, light meat	3 ounces	27

Think about this the next time you sit down to a meal: If you're having a regular hamburger on a roll for lunch, you've used up nearly half your protein for the day. If you're having a big bowlful of hearty macaroni and bean soup, you've used up only about a third of your daily protein.

How Many Grams Are Right for You?

Here's how the Anti-Aging Diet works to get you down to your ideal weight as you become healthier and more vitally alive. First, select the appropriate number of grams of protein for your goal weight.

- 50 grams of protein a day if your goal is to be between 100 and 149 pounds
- 60 grams of protein if your goal is to be between 150 and 199 pounds
- 75 grams of protein if your goal is to be between 200 and 230 pounds
- 85 grams of protein if your goal is to be over 230

(If you wish to customize your diet further, you may calculate the exact number of protein grams for your goal weight by eating 1 gram of protein for every 3 pounds of desired weight.)

The menu plans for the Anti-Aging Diet will direct you in terms of how many daily servings of carbohydrates, proteins, and fats you're allowed. When you're within five pounds of your ideal weight, you'll reach the lifetime program, on which you'll gradually increase your servings in the unlimited categories by one a week for four weeks until your weight stabilizes. If you haven't gained back any weight during this time, and if you wish to eat more servings in these categories, by all means do so.

The Balance of Protein Grams and Caloric Intake

Now, you're probably asking why a 105-pound woman should be consuming the same number of grams of protein as a 149-pound man. Because a gram is such a small amount by weight, the difference between the almost 35 grams of protein the woman needs and the 50 grams the man requires is about an ounce, so I've grouped them together in the diet. Now, here's where the element of calories comes into play, and this is about the only reason you have to understand caloric intake when you're talking about diets.

You may know that you'll lose weight if you burn more calories than you eat. When you begin any diet, you burn a combination of muscle protein, stored carbohydrates, and fat. As you continue to lose weight, the proportion of these elements changes. Because you clearly need muscle protein in order to survive, your body starts burning a higher percentage of fats. Since you no longer need the extra muscle tissue and collagen that was in place to hold up all the fat you've lost, you lose that as well. Someone with a formerly pudgy face may end up with cheekbones at the end of a diet!

Now assume the 105-pound woman and 149-pound man both have ten pounds to lose. The man will lose them first, because he has fewer fat stores to burn. In order to maintain his new weight, he'll switch to the lifetime program, thereby increasing the number of portions of different food groups he eats every day. But he will *not* increase his allotment of animal protein because 50 grams is all he needs. Therefore, the percentage of protein in his diet will go down (possibly to 10 or 12 percent of his total daily intake) as his caloric intake goes up. He'll be able to maintain his new weight and stay healthier instead of regaining the weight because he'll be eating more but better than before the Anti-Aging Diet.

The woman will take more time to lose her ten pounds. Women, as you know, are constructed for childbearing and breast-feeding with additional fat padding in the breasts, hips, and thighs. A woman's proportion of fat to lean body mass is greater than a man's. And because she's smaller, the ten pounds is a greater percentage of her body weight. But even though her weight loss will be a slower process, the dieting woman will also get down to her goal weight. And at that point she'll also switch over to the lifetime program. Though she will probably not be able to consume as many servings (and therefore as many calories) as the man, her caloric intake will rise since she's no longer dieting. By sticking with her 50-gram protein limit, however, the percentage of protein she's consuming will drop to about 10 or 12 percent of her total daily intake. But she, too, will find that she can maintain her new weight instead of regaining.

How Much Should You Weigh?

Most people know if they're overweight simply by the way their clothes fit, the way they feel, and the way they look in the mirror, regardless of the reading on their scale.

In order to be certain of just how overweight you are and how far you have to go to reach your goal, it's a good idea to find out how much of your body is fat and how much is lean muscle mass. You can learn this information by having a "pinch test" with a set of calipers (many doctors and health clubs have this device), or with a sophisticated measurement called bioelectrical impedance, in which a painless electrical impulse is sent through your body from your finger to your foot. The more fat you have, the longer it takes for the current to pass through your body because fat is an insulator and slows current down. Muscle and organs are mostly water, which conducts electricity. Your own physician may be able to perform this test in his office; if not, he'll be able to refer you to a hospital or clinic that has the equipment.

Women should have between 18 and 25 percent of body weight as fat; men should have between 12 and 18 percent. When you know your body's fat composition, you'll know how much weight you should lose and how many grams of protein a day you should be eating to lose weight.

Please take a look at the following ideal weights for men and women. I know that most weight tables offer the proverbial large frame cop-out. My feeling is that although there is an acceptable and safe range of weight depending upon your build, most people who are heavy automatically use the excuse that they're big boned. Actually, there are fewer large-framed people running around than you might think.

IDEAL WEIGHT IN POUNDS

WOMEN		MEN	
Height	Weight	Height	Weight
4'9"	102–111	5'1"	138–150
4'10"	103–113	5'2"	140–153

Women		Men	
Height	Weight	Height	Weight
4′11″	104–115	5′3″	142–156
5′0″	106–118	5′4″	144–160
5″1″	108–121	5′5″	146–164
5′2″	111–124	5′6″	149–168
5′3″	114–127	5′7″	152–172
5′4″	117–130	5′8″	155–176
5′5″	120–133	5′9″	158–180
5′6″	123–136	5′10″	161–184
5′7″	126–139	5′11″	164–188
5′8″	129–142	6′0″	168–192
5′9″	132–145	6′1″	172–197
5′10″	135–148	6′2″	176–202
5′11″	138–151	6′3″	181–207
6′0″	141–154	6′4″	186–212

The Five Food Groups

We were all taught that there were four basic food groups, and in order to achieve maximum growth as children and optimum health as adults, we were required to consume requisite amounts from each of the groups every day: meat and poultry, dairy, cereals and grains, and fruits and vegetables (usually in that order, with protein first).

Today, there's hot controversy around the issue of these food designations. One group of eminent physicians, based in Washington, D.C., is recommending that we remove meat, poultry, and dairy completely from the roster and that everyone consume them only occasionally. Most nutritionists go along with a restriction on red meat and advise removing the skin from poultry, but balk at the idea of restricting all animal protein in a normal diet.

My feeling is that we need to liberalize our groups. On the Anti-Aging Diet you'll be eating from five food groups. (Fats and sweets, you will notice, are not to be considered as part of the diet. Jam and honey will be allowed on the lifetime plan.)

1. Fruits
2. Vegetables, non-starchy and starchy
3. Cereals and grains
4. Legumes, nuts, and seeds
5. Animal products (meat, poultry, dairy)

What are legumes? They are plant-based protein foods. Legumes include lentils, peas, tofu, and tempeh (two foods made of soybeans), garbanzos (chick-peas), and every bean you can think of—kidney beans, navy beans, mung beans, adzuki beans, white beans (cannellini), limas, soybeans, and broad beans.

Nuts and seeds also fall loosely into this category because they are plant-based protein foods; however, they are very high in fat, and you should therefore limit your number of portions. Peanuts, cashews, walnuts, pignoli nuts, pistachio nuts, Brazil nuts, and sunflower, sesame, and pumpkin seeds should all be eaten in moderation.

Legumes are low-cost protein sources; they are easy to prepare and absolutely delicious (see the recipes in Chapter 12). When properly stored, they will last indefinitely on your kitchen shelves—and in glass jars they make a wonderful visual assortment, as well. But they're not intended just to be put on view—they are a positive alternative to animal protein and will become a vital part of your anti-aging diet.

Shifting the Balance of Your Meals

We have all been brought up believing that "main dishes" consist of meat, eggs, poultry, or fish and "side dishes" were vegetables and starches. On this radical, breakthrough diet it's the reverse.

In the societies where heart disease and cancer rates are far lower than ours, meats are used as side dishes or condiments, just to add a little extra taste to the meal. The reason is usually less health oriented than pocketbook oriented. A large family in a small Mexican village simply can't afford a piece of meat for every member and, in many cases, beef may not even be available. So a meal of beans and rice or corn with chilis makes up a main course here.

A Chinese stir fry might be made up of noodles and vegetables with a little pork or fish tossed in for flavor. Japanese shabu-shabu is a steamed vegetable and noodle stew with a little meat or chicken added. Couscous from North Africa is basically a delicious wheat dish garnished with lamb; spinach pies are a staple in Greece, and many South American and Native American dishes are cornmeal based. An Italian risotto is a rice dish with a few shrimp to dress it up. A Spanish paella is going to depend on what the chef has on hand—shellfish, sausage, chicken—but its main ingredient is always rice.

In America, of course, we don't have any problem with availability of ingredients. Our supermarkets fairly bulge with produce—there are typically 26,000 items in the aisles on any given day. But beef, lamb, pork, chicken, turkey, fish, or shellfish are the most expensive items in your shopping basket, and by using just a small portion in a meal, you're going to be saving hundreds of dollars a year as you shed those unwanted pounds.

From now on, protein is the extra; meat, eggs, poultry, and fish are "side dishes." Any pasta or vegetable dish now becomes your main course. You'll be getting a lot of fiber—25 to 35 grams a day—in your complex carbohydrates, which means that your digestive tract is going to start working much more efficiently. A high-fiber diet significantly lowers your risk of prostate, colon, rectal, uterine, and breast cancers. Fruit, which is full of fiber, is the best dessert or snack you can choose. You can eat all you want once you get to lifetime program.

You'll find, when you start rebalancing the food in your diet, that your dinner plate looks just as full, only the protein and fat take up much less room. Remember, the proportions of your total daily intake while you're losing weight are these:

20 percent protein; 20 percent fat; 60 percent complex carbohydrates

---

When your main goal is longevity, what's essential is to restrict protein. That's why I want you to concentrate only on how many

grams of protein you eat each day. You can pick and choose lib-
erally from the first four food groups and add on a little from the
animal products group to equal your daily gram requirements.

What About Cholesterol?

The media have picked up the issue of harmful cholesterol and
run with it. If you're health-conscious, you probably know your
cholesterol count now and realize it should be under 200 for maximum protection from coronary artery disease. You also know that
you're taking in cholesterol when you eat animal products and
saturated fats. Egg yolks, organ meats (liver and kidneys), caviar,
and shellfish are all exceedingly high in cholesterol. Butter, cream,
most soft cheeses, and other high-fat animal foods are chock full
of cholesterol. And saturated fats, like coconut and palm oil, are
converted to cholesterol in the liver.

But cholesterol itself is only half bad. It's the low-density lipo-
proteins or LDLs that allow fatty deposits to accumulate on the
interior walls of blood vessels, blocking free flow of blood to and
from the heart. You are probably aware that high density lipopro-
teins or HDLs are the "good guy" cholesterols that help to break
down fats and protect your cardiovascular system. It's been clearly
proven that you can raise your HDLs with a high-fiber diet and
exercise.

The Anti-Aging Diet will automatically take care of your cholesterol count. By reducing fats and animal proteins to 20 percent
of your daily total intake, you simply won't be eating cholesterol-
rich foods. And by eating plenty of complex carbohydrates and
getting on a daily exercise regimen (see Chapter 7), you'll be boosting your protective HDLs sky high.

What About Salt?

The current recommended daily requirement for sodium is 500
milligrams daily. Most Americans eat 4 to 6 grams, ten times that

amount. They salt their food as they prepare it and salt it again when it comes to the table.

Many people complain that "diet foods" taste dull because they're not allowed to use any salt on them. On the Anti-Aging Diet, you'll be restricting your sodium intake naturally because most of the salt you eat comes from animal protein and processed foods, from cheeses to salad dressings to cold cuts. Since the proportion of these foods in your diet is going to be small, you really don't have to worry too much about adding a little salt as you prepare your meals or adding a few grains at the table if you eliminate it in the cooking process. It is important to keep your sodium intake low, however, if you have high blood pressure. If you're hypertensive, you have increased concentrations of sodium in your tissues and tend to retain fluids. Obviously, the more salt you eat, the more sodium your body has to contend with.

But if your blood pressure is normal, you don't have to be overly concerned about how much salt you use. In addition to salt, the Anti-Aging Diet encourages you to experiment freely with other condiments in your cooking and eating. There's no reason for any food to taste dull or bland, particularly since as you extend your life span you're going to have many more years of meals ahead of you!

What About Sugar?

Sugar is a simple carbohydrate, as opposed to pasta or bread, which are complex carbohydrates. Simple sugars don't have any nutritive value, which means that when you eat sugar, you're taking in empty calories. Sugar has only 4 calories per gram, as opposed to fat, which has 9 calories per gram. If you crave that sweet taste and absolutely must satisfy your need for it, please choose a sugar-free hard candy instead of a candy bar. The hard candy will last you much longer and has none of the harmful fats in the chocolate and filling of the bar.

While you're losing weight on the Anti-Aging Diet, you'll get as much sugar as you want by eating fruit. As you move onto the lifetime program, you'll be using jam or honey on your toast. And you can eat nonfat frozen yogurt as an occasional dessert, in addition to the terrific sweet recipes in Chapter 12.

A Few Pointers for My Vegetarian Readers

Suppose you've already given up animal products in whole or in part. There are many confirmed vegetarians—like my wife, Molly—who eat no eggs, cheese, red meat, chicken, or fish. Are they automatically on the Anti-Aging Diet? Not necessarily, but they won't have to adapt their eating quite as radically as meat eaters will to get on the program.

Vegetarians may still be consuming too much protein if they still eat eggs and dairy products or even if they make up most of their meals from the legumes category. If you are a vegetarian who eats about 200 grams of beans, peanuts, tofu, eggs, or cheese a day, you must make some changes in your diet. Switch the balance of your meals to pasta, rice, vegetables, and fruit and lower the amounts of the legumes or eggs and dairy you eat and the frequency with which you eat them.

Remember, your kidneys, liver, and colon don't know the difference between animal and vegetable protein, and you can put undue stress on these organs even on a vegetarian diet if it's too high in protein.

What About Alcohol, Caffeine, and Soda?

Alcohol must be processed by your liver, your body's cleansing organ, giving it more work to do without any nutritional benefit to your body. And alcohol slows your reflexes, makes your eyes bloodshot and your skin puffy and taxes your heart. The leading causes of ulcer diseases are alcohol abuse and smoking. In Japan, the many fatal cases of stomach cancer have been linked to excessive consumption of alcohol and the excessive use of tobacco.

I'd like you to give up alcohol completely. It's a drug, like any other recreational drug, and it's addictive. You may think you need that drink at the end of the day to unwind, but a two-mile walk would relax you far better and leave you feeling clear headed and refreshed. But if you simply can't comply with complete elimination of alcohol in your diet, at least give it up for the period of time when you're losing the weight. Since alcohol loosens your inhibitions, you may find it difficult to stick to a diet if you have a few drinks before or during your meal.

When you switch to the lifetime program, you may have one four-ounce drink a week of beer or wine. At no time, however, should you exceed three drinks a week on this program.

Caffeine is hard on the bones and constricts the blood vessels. It's been implicated as an exacerbating factor in premenstrual syndrome. And since caffeine affects the central nervous system, it can be responsible for mood swings that might interfere with your compliance with a diet and exercise program. Believe me, you won't need any more artificial stimulants because of the increased energy you'll have from being on the Anti-Aging Diet.

Soda frequently has as much caffeine as coffee or tea, and it also contains phosphates that can interfere with the acid-alkaline balance of the blood.

So what do you drink? Your first choice should be water—at least eight to ten eight-ounce glasses a day. Water is a wonderful thirst quencher, it's filling, and it's essential for cleansing excess protein from your body.

You may also drink vegetable and fruit juices, a flavored seltzer, or a juice-and-seltzer combination drink. Herbal tea is great at all times of day or night.

Vitamins and Minerals—Critical Foods for Maximum Health

While you're busy learning about new foods and new food combinations from the menu plans, I want you to consider a daily dose of twelve critical foods that are particularly rich in vitamins and minerals. These foods can make the difference for you between simply losing weight and feeling better and living a longer, more disease free life. There is new research indicating that these foods may actually inhibit some early cellular mutations that may lead to certain cancers.

In Chapter 8, I'll explain why vitamin and mineral supplementation can make such a difference in the preservation of good health and in slowing the aging process. But for now, let's just think about the critical foods that provide you with the vital nutrients, which I call "golden ones":

- Vitamin C, beta carotene, vitamin E, and selenium are all antioxidants that slow the aging process and reduce the risk of cancer and heart disease
- Chromium reduces the risk of cancer and of diabetes
- Iron prevents anemia
- Capsaicin reduces the risk of cancer
- Fiber reduces the risk of colon cancer by increasing the activity of natural detoxifying enzymes that help the body to clear out toxins and enhance the immune system

You might want to think about eating one of the foods that contain these nutrients each day as an extra vitamin supplement.

The Essential Anti-Aging Foods

Here is your list of essential foods. They are easy to fit into your diet, and there's something on the list for every palate, even if you're a picky eater. They offer some of the best protection your supermarket dollars can buy. Eat one of these foods every day to boost the amount of essential nutrients:

1. Broccoli contains vitamin C and beta carotene
2. Canteloupe contains beta carotene
3. Carrots are high in beta carotene
4. Garlic is rich in selenium
5. Nuts are, in moderation, rich in chromium
6. Olive oil supplies vitamin E
7. Papaya is rich in vitamin C
8. Prunes are high in chromium and iron
9. Red chili peppers provide vitamin A, capsaicin
10. Romaine lettuce and other green, leafy vegetables have folate (B-vitamin) and chromium
11. Spinach has beta carotene and iron
12. Wheat germ provides vitamin E

A Few Good Words About Modified Fasting

Fasting is one of the oldest personal practices known to man. It has been used in religion, as a means of individual political protest, and as a moral exercise in learning. It has also been badly abused as a means of weight loss.

I am *not* advocating fasting as a way to squeeze yourself into your size eight jeans or a dress for that wedding that's coming up in a week. This is a terrible way to look at the dieting process and can be ultimately harmful. A generation of anorexic young women who are overly concerned about the size of their bodies has suffered greatly from the fasting process.

But for normal, healthy individuals, I *do* recommend a modified fast on juice or my Back-to-Basics Soup (see page 85). On the Anti-Aging Diet, for however long it takes you to get within five pounds of your ideal weight, I would like you to fast one day a week. You will find that the high vitamin and mineral content of my Back-to-Basics Soup will energize you, both the day you're fasting and for several days after.

When you reach the lifetime program, you'll implement the soup fast once every few weeks if you like, again, to allow your body time to rest and to give yourself an extra energy boost. I think you'll enjoy its benefits so much that you'll decide to keep using it.

If the idea of fasting is completely foreign to you, and you feel you just can't, I won't insist. But most of my patients, however reluctant they were initially, were surprised at the ease with which they incorporated a fast into their diet. They said that it really put them in touch with their bodies. I very strongly recommend that you try it just once before ruling it out entirely. Cutting your food consumption for a day gives your body a real chance to rest and gives your digestive tract the opportunity to cleanse itself of toxins.

A day of fasting is in no way harmful *if* you're not pregnant or nursing, and *if* you're not suffering from a severely debilitating illness such as congestive heart failure, pneumonia, an acute viral condition, or metastatic cancer. Teenagers, also, should *not* fast because they are still going through an important developmental growth stage.

Fasting every once in a while gives you a new perception about the way your body reacts to hunger. You *think* you need a big meal three times a day because you always eat them three times a day. *Not* eating shows you where your real hunger is. You may be very surprised about how energized you feel when you don't have a full stomach.

As you reeducate your body toward accepting a diet high in complex carbohydrates, and as you wean yourself off the heavy protein and fat diet you used to consume, you can also teach your body to utilize its new energy stores with a one-day fast for a real boost.

I'd like you to drink up to 16 ounces of fluid—either Back-to-Basics Soup or vegetable juices—three times daily on your one-day fast. If you're prone to hypoglycemia, you should drink 8 ounces of soup six times a day instead.

If you experience lightheadedness or nausea during your day of fasting, be sure to eat a few low-salt crackers and have a small amount of your next portion of soup.

Back-to-Basics Soup

2 ounces onions, cut into eighths
4 ounces carrots, coarsely chopped
2 ounces fresh spinach leaves, well washed and drained, coarsely chopped
4 ounces broccoli flowerettes

2 cups water
2 cloves garlic, peeled and crushed
1/4 teaspoon freshly ground black pepper
1/4 teaspoon salt
1/2 teaspoon paprika
1 28-ounce can tomatoes without salt

Place the raw vegetables in a food processor and process until finely chopped. Put the vegetables into a Dutch oven or 6-cup saucepan, add the water, garlic, seasonings, and tomatoes. Bring to a boil, then lower heat and simmer, uncovered, until the carrots are tender, about 20 minutes. Do not overcook. Serve cold or hot.

Yields: 6 servings
Serving size: 1 cup
Calories per serving: 46

Grams of protein per serving: 2
Grams of fat per serving: 0.5
Milligrams of sodium per serving: 333

THE TWO-STAGE DIET:

Weight Loss and Lifetime Program

FIRST STAGE: WEIGHT LOSS

The Anti-Aging Diet is for weight loss and cleansing, and also for setting new goals for exercise and creating a more positive attitude toward your commitment to anti-aging.

During this first stage, your body is going to go through a real catharsis as it begins to detoxify. By lowering your protein intake and shifting your food balance, you'll be losing weight as you give your body a needed rest. You'll be boosting your immune system by the addition of protective foods and allowing your kidneys and liver the opportunity to do less work and, ultimately, recover from years of processing too much protein.

On the first day of the Anti-Aging Diet, you'll be eating the same foods as you're allowed during the lifetime program. The beauty of my breakthrough diet is that you're not doing anything unusual to lose weight. All you're doing is reapportioning the types of foods on your plate.

First find your ideal weight (see page 74) in the listing below, which will give you the appropriate number of grams of protein you should consume each day.

- 50 grams for 100 to 149 pounds
- 60 grams for 150 to 199 pounds
- 75 grams for 200 to 229 pounds
- 85 grams for over 230 pounds

(You may also customize your diet for a better "fit." Simply determine the exact number of grams of protein you need by using the formula of **1 gram of protein for every 3 pounds of desired weight.**)

Then use the Sample 7-Day Menu Plan (pages 89–116) that applies to you—for 50, 60, 75, or 85 grams of protein per day. For the first three weeks, keep an accurate count of how many grams of protein you eat using the calculations in the menu plans. This is a good way to educate yourself about how much protein you're getting from the foods you eat. Don't worry about caloric intake— really! Just try to hit your gram allowance as indicated above. If you go above it one day, don't worry too much—you can always make up for it the next.

I want you to be an active participant in your own healthful eating program, rather than a slavish follower of a rigid set of rules. Once you've learned to use the Anti-Aging Diet menus for weight loss, you'll be able to create your own favorite meals. When you are ready, consult the Protein Intake Chart in the Creative Menu Planner (pages 118–122) that applies to your protein intake need. These charts list the number of servings allowed daily for each food group. By consulting the Protein Gram Counters (pages 123–130) you can determine the serving size and calculate the grams of protein you should be consuming to maintain your daily protein intake need—50, 60, 75, or 85 grams per day.

Be sure to drink at least ten 8-ounce glasses of water or other liquids a day.

The Anti-Aging Diet takes about three weeks for most people. However, if you have significantly more weight to lose, do not move on to the lifetime program until you're within 5 pounds of your goal. If you had 10 pounds or less to lose when you started the diet, after three weeks you may move on to the lifetime program.

Crossing the Last Plateau: Those Final Five Pounds

I have never, ever met a woman who didn't tell me that she needed to lose just five more pounds. No matter how successful she's been on her diet, she just can't manage to take off that final five. Some patients find that drinking more water accelerates the loss of those last pounds. Others tell me that, as hard as they try, they just can't do it.

Hitting a plateau is natural as your metabolism reaches a level at which it can comfortably function and from which it doesn't want to move. The problem with reaching a plateau (and everyone does during the weight loss process—men and women) is that it's a real downer. You feel all your commitment and motivation haven't been enough, that there are elements outside your control holding you back from reaching your true goal. And then you may lose the spirit and stop trying.

I don't want you to think this way about your weight. Remember that the Anti-Aging Diet is not a quick fix. It is a revolutionary, ongoing process that is not just making you thinner but making you healthier in the long run. You have all your life to lose those last 5 pounds. And even on a plateau, when you're not losing, you're boosting your immune system, protecting yourself from chronic disease, and adding energy to your days and years to your life.

However, I can understand the longing for that final confirmation that you've arrived. And you *can* lose the last 5 pounds. Really!

In order to get off your plateau and start losing again, simply double your exercise program for thirty days and do a juice fast every fourth day. You should drink any combination of low-salt vegetable juices and fruit juices to equal 16 ounces of juice four times a day and at least four to six 8–ounce glasses of water per day. This technique will take those extra pounds off most people.

But some bodies are more stubborn than others. If you find that you are *still* having trouble, I want you to try the Anti-Aging five-pound crisis intervention program:

1. Day one: juice fast, 16 ounces four times a day
2. Day two: solid vegetables (raw, boiled, or baked)
3. Day three: Back-to-Basics Soup
   On the fourth day you will return to your lifetime eating plan.

You can repeat this program up to four times monthly or until the final 5 pounds have been shed. **This crisis intervention program should never be followed if you are ill or if you are suffering from any serious disease such as diabetes, heart disease, or cancer. If you are in any doubt as to whether you should follow this program, consult with your own physician.**

Anti-Aging Weight-Loss Diet
Sample 7-Day Menu Plans

50 Grams per Day Protein Intake (1000 Calories)
(For desired weight range 100–149 pounds)

DAY 1

			Grams	
SERVING SIZE	FOOD	CALORIES	PROTEIN	FAT
	Breakfast			
¾ cup	oatmeal	100	5	2
1 teaspoon	sugar or honey (if desired)	16	0	0
½ cup	skim milk	50	4	0
1	orange	60	0	0
	Lunch			
2 servings	Vegetable "Tea"*	142	4	0
½	whole wheat bagel	80	2	1
1 table-spoon	reduced-fat cream cheese	60	3	5
	Snacks—may be enjoyed anytime during the day or evening			
2	fresh fruits	120	0	0
½ cup	skim milk	50	4	0
	Dinner			
1 serving	Fish Naranja*	126	17	1
½ cup	Wild Risotto*	104	4	3
1 cup	steamed broccoli spears	50	4	0
1 teaspoon	olive oil	45	0	5
1 teaspoon	lemon juice (if desired)			
1 cup	no-salt vegetable juice	25	2	0
	TOTALS:	1028	49	17

*Recipes given in this book.

DAY 2

SERVING SIZE	FOOD	CALORIES	Grams	
			PROTEIN	FAT
	Breakfast			
1 serving	Mollen Shake*	132	8	1
1 slice	whole grain toast	80	2	1
1 teaspoon	Reduced-fat margarine (if desired)	15	0	2
	Lunch			
1 serving	Fennel and Watercress Salad with Blood Oranges and Pecans*	241	7	17
1 cup	no-salt tomato juice	25	2	0
	Snacks—may be enjoyed anytime during the day or evening			
2	fresh fruits	120	0	0
	Dinner			
1 cup	Lentil and Brown Rice Soup*	183	10	1
1 serving	Jalapeño-Honey Cornbread*	144	4	4
1 teaspoon	honey (if desired)	16	0	0
1 cup	skim milk	100	8	0
	TOTALS:	1056	41	26

*Recipes given in this book.

DAY 3

SERVING SIZE	FOOD	CALORIES	Grams PROTEIN	FAT
Breakfast				
½ cup	High-fiber ready-to-eat cereal	70	4	1
1 cup	skim milk	100	8	0
½	banana	60	0	0
1 cup	Herbal tea (if desired)	0	0	0
Lunch				
1½ cups	pasta	250	6	1
½ cup	Marinara Sauce*	77	2	3
1 small	tossed green salad	25	2	0
1 table-spoon	reduced-fat dressing	20	0	1
Snacks—may be enjoyed anytime during the day or evening				
2	fresh fruits	120	0	0
Dinner				
1 serving	Christopher's Fish Soup*	243	23	7
1 slice	sourdough bread	80	3	0
	TOTALS:	1045	48	13

*Recipes given in this book.

DAY 4

				Grams	
SERVING SIZE	FOOD	CALORIES	PROTEIN	FAT

Breakfast

¾ cup	Wheatena	100	4	0
1 teaspoon	sugar or honey (if desired)	16	0	0
½ cup	skim milk	50	4	0
1	orange	60	0	0

Lunch

2 servings	Sesame Pasta Salad*	186	9	8
1 cup	no-salt vegetable juice	25	2	0
1 cup	fresh melon chunks	60	0	0

Snacks—may be enjoyed anytime during the day or evening

2	fresh fruits	120	0	0

Dinner

1 serving	Christopher's Fish Soup*	324	30	9
1 cup	no-salt vegetable juice	25	2	0
	TOTALS:	966	51	17

*Recipe given in this book.

DAY 5

SERVING SIZE	FOOD	CALORIES	Grams	
			PROTEIN	FAT
Breakfast				
¾ cup	oatmeal	100	5	2
1 teaspoon	sugar or honey (if desired)	16	0	0
½ cup	skim milk	50	4	0
1	orange or other citrus fruit	60	0	0
Lunch				
2 servings	Back-to-Basics Soup*	92	4	1
2 slices	whole grain bread	160	4	2
½ cup	skim milk	50	4	0
Snacks—may be enjoyed anytime during the day or evening				
2	fresh fruits	120	0	0
Dinner				
½ serving	Penne with Tomato, Basil, and Garlic Sauce*	200	7	1
1 serving	Squash and Apple Bake*	124	2	2
1 small	tossed green salad	25	2	0
1 tablespoon	reduced-fat dressing	20	0	1
	TOTALS:	1017	32	9

*Recipes given in this book.

DAY 6

SERVING SIZE	FOOD	CALORIES	Grams PROTEIN	FAT
Breakfast				
½ cup	high-fiber ready-to-eat cereal	70	4	1
1 cup	skim milk	100	8	0
1	orange	60	0	0
Lunch				
1	Very Important Potato V.I.P.*	262	12	1
1 cup	no-salt vegetable juice	25	2	0
1 cup	fresh raw vegetables	25	2	0
Snacks—may be enjoyed anytime during the day or evening				
2	fresh fruits	120	0	0
Dinner				
3 servings	Fish Naranja*	126	17	1
1 cup	pasta or rice	160	4	1
	TOTALS:	1001	50	4

*Recipes given in this book.

DAY 7

			Grams	
SERVING SIZE	FOOD	CALORIES	PROTEIN	FAT
Breakfast				
1 serving	Ricottacakes*	155	12	5
1 cup	fresh berries or sliced cinnamon-flavored apples	60	0	0
1 table-spoon	Lite syrup (if desired)	25	0	0
Lunch				
2 servings	Vegetable "Tea"*	142	4	0
1 cup	nonfat plain yogurt	100	12	0
1	whole wheat roll	80	2	1

Snacks—may be enjoyed anytime during the day or evening

2	fresh fruits	120	0	0

Dinner

1 serving	Tortilla Pizza with Stir Fry Veggies and Black Bean Sauce*	343	18	12
	TOTALS:	1025	48	18

*Recipes given in this book.

60 GRAMS PER DAY PROTEIN INTAKE (1200 CALORIES)
(For desired weight range 150–199 pounds)
DAY 1

serving size	food	calories	Grams protein	fat
Breakfast				
1 serving	Mollen Shake*	132	8	1
1	English muffin	140	4	1
1 table-spoon	unsweetened apple butter	30	0	0
Lunch				
1 serving	Christopher's Fish Soup*	324	30	9
1 cup	no-salt vegetable juice	25	2	0
Snacks—may be enjoyed anytime during the day or evening				
3	fresh fruits	180	0	0
3 cups	air-popped popcorn	100	3	0
1 serving	Zucchini-Mushroom Lasagne*	161	9	6
1 serving	Almond Broccoli*	60	3	4
1 serving	Fiery Tomatoes*	61	2	1
	TOTALS:	1213	61	22

*Recipes given in this book.

DAY 2

SERVING SIZE	FOOD	CALORIES	Grams	
			PROTEIN	FAT
Breakfast				
¾ cup	oatmeal	100	5	2
1 teaspoon	sugar or honey (if desired)	16	0	0
½ cup	skim milk	50	4	0
1	orange	60	0	0
Lunch				
2 ounces	sliced turkey breast	100	16	2
2 slices	whole grain bread	160	4	2
2 teaspoons	mustard (if desired)	10	1	1
1 serving	Oriental Cabbage Salad*	34	2	0
Snacks—may be enjoyed anytime during the day or evening				
3	fresh fruits	180	0	0
Dinner				
1½ servings	Black Bean Cowboy Stew*	324	24	5
1 slice	whole grain toast	80	2	1
1 teaspoon	garlic-flavored reduced-fat margarine	15	0	2
1 small	tossed green salad	25	2	0
1 tablespoon	reduced-fat dressing	20	0	1
	TOTALS:	1174	60	16

*Recipes given in this book.

DAY 3

			Grams	
SERVING SIZE	FOOD	CALORIES	PROTEIN	FAT
	Breakfast			
1 serving	Ricottacakes*	155	12	5
1 cup	fresh berries or sliced cinnamon-flavored apples	60	0	0
1 table-spoon	Lite syrup (if desired)	25	0	0
	Lunch			
1 serving	Linguini with Broccoli Sauce*	331	13	5
1 cup	fresh melon chunks	60	0	0
	Snacks—*may be enjoyed anytime during the day or evening*			
3	fresh fruits	180	0	0
	Dinner			
1 serving	Foil-Baked Citrus Sea Bass*	173	31	1
1 cup	pasta or rice	160	4	1
½ cup	stewed tomatoes	25	2	0
	TOTALS:	1169	62	12

*Recipes given in this book.

DAY 4

SERVING SIZE	FOOD	CALORIES	Grams PROTEIN	FAT
	Breakfast			
1 serving	Mollen Shake*	132	8	1
1 slice	whole grain toast	80	2	1
1 cup	Herbal Tea* (if desired)	0	0	0
	Lunch			
1 serving	Black Bean Cowboy Stew*	216	16	3
1 serving	Jalapeño-Honey Cornbread*	144	4	4
1 teaspoon	honey (if desired)	16	0	0
1 cup	skim milk	100	8	0
	Snack—may be enjoyed anytime during the day or evening			
3	fresh fruits	180	0	0
	Dinner			
1 serving	Fish Naranja*	126	17	1
1 cup	rice	200	4	0
½ cup	fresh green beans	25	2	0
1 small	tossed green salad	25	2	0
1 tablespoon	reduced-fat dressing	20	0	1
	TOTALS:	1264	63	11

*Recipes given in this book.

DAY 5

SERVING SIZE	FOOD	CALORIES	Grams PROTEIN	FAT

Breakfast

SERVING SIZE	FOOD	CALORIES	PROTEIN	FAT
½ cup	high-fiber ready-to-eat cereal	70	4	1
1 cup	skim milk	100	8	0
1	orange	60	0	0

Lunch

1½ cups	Lentil and Brown Rice Soup*	274	15	2
1 slice	sourdough bread	80	3	0
1 cup	no-salt vegetable juice	25	2	0

Snacks—may be enjoyed anytime during the day or evening

3	fresh fruits	180	0	0

Dinner

4 ounces	Broiled Marinated Shrimp*	216	23	5
½ cup	baked yam	100	2	0
1 small	tossed green salad	25	2	0
2 tablespoons	Vinaigrette dressing	50	0	5
	TOTALS:	1180	59	13

*Recipes given in this book.

DAY 6

SERVING SIZE	FOOD	CALORIES	Grams PROTEIN	FAT
Breakfast				
1	bagel	160	4	2
1 table-spoon	reduced-fat cream cheese	60	3	5
1 table-spoon	unsweetened apple butter	30	0	0
1	orange	60	0	0
Lunch				
1 serving	Linguini with Broccoli Sauce*	331	13	5
1 cup	skim milk	100	8	0
Snacks—may be enjoyed anytime during the day or evening				
3	fresh fruits	180	0	0
Dinner				
1 serving	Chicken Chalupa*	273	24	2
¼ cup	Fresh Salsa* or Salsa Pronto*	20	1	0
	TOTALS:	1214	53	14

*Recipes given in this book.

DAY 7

SERVING SIZE	FOOD	CALORIES	Grams	
			PROTEIN	FAT
Breakfast				
1 serving	Mollen Shake*	132	8	1
1	English muffin	140	4	1
1 table-spoon	peanut butter	90	5	7
Lunch				
1 serving	Sesame Pasta Salad*	186	9	8
1 cup	no-salt vegetable juice	25	2	0
1 cup	fresh melon chunks	60	0	0
Snacks—may be enjoyed anytime during the day or evening				
3	fresh fruits	180	0	0
Dinner				
1 serving	Apple Salmon and Sauerkraut en Papillotte*	361	33	19
5 ounces	boiled red-skinned potatoes	150	4	0
	TOTALS:	1324	65	36

*Recipes given in this book.

75 Grams per Day Protein Intake (1500 Calories)
(For desired weight range 200–229 pounds)

DAY 1

			Grams	
SERVING SIZE	FOOD	CALORIES	PROTEIN	FAT

Breakfast

½ cup	high-fiber ready-to-eat cereal	70	4	1
1 cup	skim milk	100	8	0
1	orange	60	0	0

Lunch

2 servings	Red and Yellow Bell Pepper Soup*	236	10	8
2 slices	whole grain bread	160	4	2
2 table-spoons	unsweetened apple butter	60	0	0

Snacks—may be enjoyed anytime during the day or evening

| 4 | fresh fruits | 240 | 0 | 0 |
| 1 cup | nonfat plain yogurt | 100 | 12 | 0 |

Dinner

1 serving	Lemon Garlic Chicken Paillards*	372	40	10
1 small	tossed green salad	25	2	0
2 table-spoons	reduced-fat dressing	40	0	2
1 slice	French bread	80	2	0
	TOTALS:	1543	82	23

*Recipes given in this book.

DAY 2

SERVING SIZE	FOOD	CALORIES	Grams PROTEIN	FAT

Breakfast

SERVING SIZE	FOOD	CALORIES	PROTEIN	FAT
¾ cup	oatmeal	100	5	2
1 teaspoon	sugar or honey (if desired)	16	0	0
½ cup	skim milk	50	4	0
1	orange	60	0	0

Lunch

SERVING SIZE	FOOD	CALORIES	PROTEIN	FAT
1	Very Important Potato V.I.P.*	262	12	1
2 cups	no-salt vegetable juice	50	4	0

Snacks—may be enjoyed anytime during the day or evening

SERVING SIZE	FOOD	CALORIES	PROTEIN	FAT
4	fresh fruits	240	0	0
1	bagel	160	4	2
1 tablespoon	reduced-fat cream cheese	60	3	5

Dinner

SERVING SIZE	FOOD	CALORIES	PROTEIN	FAT
2 cups	Thai Noodles*	484	36	12
2 servings	Oriental Cabbage Salad*	68	4	0
	TOTALS:	1550	72	20

*Recipes given in this book.

DAY 3

		Calories	Grams	
SERVING SIZE	FOOD	CALORIES	PROTEIN	FAT
	Breakfast			
1 serving	Ricottacakes*	155	12	5
2 table-spoons	Lite syrup (if desired)	50	0	0
1 cup	fresh melon chunks	60	0	0
	Lunch			
1 serving	Zucchini-Mushroom Lasagne*	161	9	6
1 cup	no-salt vegetable juice	25	2	0
	Snacks—may be enjoyed anytime during the day or evening			
4	fresh fruits	240	0	0
1	bagel	160	4	2
1 table-spoon	reduced-fat cream cheese	60	3	5
	Dinner			
1 serving	Herbed Red Snapper*	164	27	6
1 serving	Neapolitan Potato Salad*	183	4	9
1 cup	stewed tomatoes	50	4	0
1	whole wheat roll	80	2	1
1 serving	Native American Pineapple Roast*	78	0	0
	TOTALS:	1499	67	34

*Recipes given in this book.

DAY 4

SERVING SIZE	FOOD	CALORIES	Grams PROTEIN	FAT
	Breakfast			
1 serving	Mollen Shake*	132	8	1
1	bagel	160	4	2
	Lunch			
1½ cups	Lentil and Brown Rice Soup*	274	15	2
1 slice	sourdough bread	80	3	0
	Snacks—may be enjoyed anytime during the day or evening			
4	fresh fruits	240	0	0
1 cup	nonfat plain yogurt	100	12	0
	Dinner			
1 serving	Penne with Tomato, Basil, and Garlic Sauce*	401	14	2
1 small	tossed green salad	25	2	0
1 tablespoon	reduced-fat dressing	20	0	1
1 cup	skim milk	100	8	0
	TOTALS:	1532	66	8

*Recipes given in this book.

DAY 5

	SERVING SIZE	FOOD	CALORIES	Grams PROTEIN	FAT

Breakfast

1 serving	Ricottacakes*	155	12	5
1 cup	fresh berries or sliced cinnamon-flavored apples	60	0	0
2 table-spoons	lite syrup (if desired)	50	0	0

Lunch

2 servings	Vegetable "Tea"*	142	4	0
1	fresh fruit	60	0	0

Snacks—may be enjoyed anytime during the day or evening

3	fresh fruits	180	0	0
1	English muffin	140	4	1
1 table-spoon	peanut butter	90	5	7

Dinner

1½ servings	Chicken Chalupa*	406	36	3
¾ cup	Fresh Salsa* or Salsa Pronto*	60	3	0
1 cup	skim milk	100	8	0
	TOTALS:	1443	72	16

*Recipes given in this book.

DAY 6

SERVING SIZE	FOOD	CALORIES	Grams PROTEIN	FAT

Breakfast

SERVING SIZE	FOOD	CALORIES	PROTEIN	FAT
1 serving	Mollen Shake*	132	8	1
1	bagel	160	4	2
2 table-spoons	unsweetened apple butter	60	0	0

Lunch

3 ounces	sliced turkey breast	150	24	3
2 slices	whole grain bread	160	4	2
2 teaspoons	mustard (if desired)	10	1	1
2 cups	no-salt vegetable juice	50	4	0

Snacks—may be enjoyed anytime during the day or evening

4	fresh fruits	240	0	0
½ cup	nonfat plain yogurt	50	6	0

Dinner

1 serving	Black Bean Cowboy Stew*	216	16	3
1 serving	Jalapeño-Honey Cornbread*	144	4	4
2 teaspoons	honey (if desired)	32	0	0
2 teaspoons	reduced-fat margarine	30	0	4
1 cup	skim milk	100	8	0
	TOTALS:	1534	79	20

*Recipes given in this book.

DAY 7

SERVING SIZE	FOOD	CALORIES	Grams PROTEIN	FAT
	Breakfast			
½ cup	high-fiber ready-to-eat cereal	70	4	1
1 cup	skim milk	100	8	0
	Lunch			
2 servings	Huevos Rancheros (Ranch-Style Eggs)*	482	30	22
1 cup	lettuce and tomato garnish	25	2	0
1 cup	fresh melon chunks	60	0	0
	Snacks—may be enjoyed anytime during the day or evening			
4	fresh fruits	240	0	0
1 cup	nonfat plain yogurt	100	12	0
	Dinner			
1 serving	Linguini with Broccoli Sauce*	331	13	5
2 cups	no-salt vegetable juice	50	4	0
	TOTALS:	1458	73	28

*Recipes given in this book.

85 GRAMS PER DAY PROTEIN INTAKE (1800 CALORIES)
(For desired weight range over 230 pounds)
DAY 1

				Grams	
SERVING SIZE		FOOD	CALORIES	PROTEIN	FAT
		Breakfast			
2	servings	Mollen Shake*	264	16	2
1	serving	Christopher's Fish Soup*	324	30	9
1	large	tossed green salad	75	6	0
3	table-spoons	reduced-fat dressing	60	0	3
		Snacks—may be enjoyed anytime during the day or evening			
5		fresh fruits	300	0	0
1		bagel	160	4	2
1	table-spoon	reduced-fat cream cheese	60	3	5
		Dinner			
1	serving	Whole Wheat Pasta with Fresh Tomato and Basil Sauce*	354	11	6
1	cup	steamed broccoli	50	4	0
1	slice	garlic toast brushed with	80	2	1
1	teaspoon	olive oil	45	0	5
1	cup	skim milk	100	8	0
		TOTALS:	1872	84	33

*Recipes given in this book.

DAY 2

			Grams	
SERVING SIZE	FOOD	CALORIES	PROTEIN	FAT

Breakfast

3	pancakes	300	6	5
2 table-spoons	lite syrup (if desired)	50	0	0
1	banana	120	0	0

Lunch

3 ounces	sliced turkey breast	150	24	3
2 slices	whole grain bread	160	4	2
2 teaspoons	mustard (if desired)	10	1	1

Snacks—may be enjoyed anytime during the day or evening

4	fresh fruits	240	0	0
3 cups	air-popped popcorn	100	3	0

Dinner

1½ servings	Lentils and Wheat Berry Ossobucco*	508	43	17
1 large	tossed green salad	75	6	0
3 table-spoons	reduced-fat dressing	60	0	3
	TOTALS:	1773	87	31

*Recipes given in this book.

DAY 3

			Grams	
SERVING SIZE	FOOD	CALORIES	PROTEIN	FAT

Breakfast

1 serving	Wheatena	100	4	0
1 teaspoon	sugar or honey	16	0	0
1	orange	60	0	0
1	bagel	160	4	2

Lunch

2 cups	Lentil and Brown Rice Soup*	366	20	3
1 cup	skim milk	100	8	0

Snacks—may be enjoyed anytime during the day or evening

3	fresh fruits	180	0	0
1 ounce	low-fat cheese	90	8	6
1 slice	whole grain bread	80	2	1

Dinner

1 serving	Red and Yellow Bell Pepper Soup*	118	5	4
1 serving	Grilled Shrimp Salad with Frizzled Tortillas*	442	29	30
2 cups	fresh melon chunks	120	0	0
	TOTALS:	1832	80	46

*Recipes given in this book.

DAY 4

SERVING SIZE	FOOD	CALORIES	Grams PROTEIN	FAT

Breakfast

SERVING SIZE	FOOD	CALORIES	PROTEIN	FAT
3	pancakes	300	6	5
1 cup	fresh berries	60	0	0
2 table-spoons	Lite syrup (if desired)	50	0	0

Lunch

1 serving	Fennel and Watercress Salad with Blood Oranges and Pecans*	241	7	17
1 slice	whole grain bread	80	2	1
2 ounces	water-packed tuna	100	16	2
1 table-spoon	reduced-fat salad dressing	20	0	1

Snacks—may be enjoyed anytime during the day or evening

5	fresh fruits	300	0	0
1 cup	nonfat plain yogurt	100	12	0

Dinner

1 serving	Grilled Chicken Breasts with Couscous Salad*	423	24	16
1 serving	Squash and Apple Bake*	124	2	2
1 cup	no-salt vegetable juice	25	2	0
	TOTALS:	1823	71	44

*Recipes given in this book.

DAY 5

SERVING SIZE	FOOD	CALORIES	Grams	
			PROTEIN	FAT
Breakfast				
1 serving	Mollen Shake*	132	8	1
1	bagel	160	4	2
1 table-spoon	reduced-fat cream cheese	60	3	5
1 table-spoon	unsweetened apple butter	30	0	0
Lunch				
½ cup	vegetarian refried beans	100	7	2
1	flour tortilla	100	3	1
1 ounce	shredded low-fat cheese	90	8	6
2 cups	shredded lettuce	50	4	0
¼ cup	Fresh Salsa* or Pronto Salsa*	20	1	0
1 cup	fresh melon chunks	60	0	0
Snacks—may be enjoyed anytime during the day or evening				
3	fresh fruits	180	0	0
3 cups	air-popped popcorn	100	3	0
1 cup	nonfat plain yogurt	100	12	0
Dinner				
1 serving	Grilled Breast of Chicken with Jicama and Sweet Peppers in Sherry Wine Vinegar Sauce*	343	25	18
1½ cups	pasta or rice	240	6	2
1 cup	steamed zucchini	50	4	0
	TOTALS:	1805	88	37

*Recipes given in this book.

DAY 6

			Grams	
SERVING SIZE	FOOD	CALORIES	PROTEIN	FAT

Breakfast

SERVING SIZE	FOOD	CALORIES	PROTEIN	FAT
2 servings	Ricottacakes*	310	24	10
1 cup	fresh berries	60	0	0
2 table-spoons	Lite syrup (if desired)	50	0	0

Lunch

SERVING SIZE	FOOD	CALORIES	PROTEIN	FAT
1 serving	Whole Wheat Pasta with Fresh Tomato and Basil Sauce*	354	11	6
1 slice	garlic toast brushed with	80	2	1
1 teaspoon	olive oil	45	0	5
1 cup	skim milk	100	8	0

Snacks—may be enjoyed anytime during the day or evening

SERVING SIZE	FOOD	CALORIES	PROTEIN	FAT
3	fresh fruits	180	0	0
1	bagel	160	4	2

Dinner

SERVING SIZE	FOOD	CALORIES	PROTEIN	FAT
1½ servings	Grilled Chicken Caesar Salad*	285	30	13
2	bread sticks	80	2	1
1 cup	no-salt vegetable juice	25	2	0
2 cups	fresh melon chunks	120	0	0
	TOTALS:	1849	83	38

*Recipes given in this book.

DAY 7

SERVING SIZE	FOOD	CALORIES	Grams PROTEIN	FAT

Breakfast

SERVING SIZE	FOOD	CALORIES	PROTEIN	FAT
½ cup	high-fiber ready-to-eat cereal	70	4	1
1 cup	skim milk	100	8	0
1 cup	orange juice	120	0	0
1 slice	whole grain toast	80	2	1
1 table-spoon	peanut butter	90	5	7

Lunch

1 serving	Linguini with Broccoli Sauce*	331	13	5
2 cups	no-salt vegetable juice	50	4	0

Snacks—may be enjoyed anytime during the day or evening

4	fresh fruits	240	0	0
3 cups	air-popped popcorn	100	3	0

Dinner

1 serving	Foil-Baked Citrus Sea Bass*	173	31	1
2 servings	Neapolitan Potato Salad*	366	8	18
1 cup	fresh green beans	50	4	0
	TOTALS:	1770	82	33

*Recipes given in this book.

SECOND STAGE:
LIFETIME PROGRAM
(The Rest of Your Life)

The second stage of the diet is the lifetime program for preventing disease, further strengthening your immune system, and maintaining your body as a finely tuned, efficient machine. It's also for setting priorities about your exercise goals and possibly for making some additional life-style changes that will enable you to live longer and better.

Your heart, kidneys, liver, and bones are all feeling the good effects of your low-protein program. You may wish to see your physician at this point for a complete physical exam and possibly to discuss a reduction in any medications you've been taking.

As you feel better and stronger, you will find that you are motivated to make decisions—physical, mental, and emotional—that have been exceptionally hard for you up until now. You may finally find the will to stop smoking, to take a stress-reduction course, to pursue a new hobby or endeavor.

You're now within five pounds of your own ideal weight. Doesn't it feel wonderful to accomplish what you've always wanted to? And it just gets better from here.

You can create your own low-protein eating plans by using the Creative Menu Planners and Protein Gram Counters that follow. Your delicious recipes can be found in Part IV.

Enjoy yourself! This is your invitation to a wonderful life-style!

Anti-Aging Creative
Menu Planners

Weight Loss and Lifetime Program

The following Protein Intake Charts show the number of servings allowed for each food group while you are on the weight-loss stage of the Anti-Aging Diet and, when you are within 5 pounds of your weight goal, the Lifetime Program you should follow. *Unlimited* means you can eat more servings in a certain category, as long as you're maintaining your ideal weight ("meet needs"); however, if you find that you're gaining, you've exceeded your needs and should drop down a serving. Increase your servings in the unlimited categories by one a week for four weeks until your weight stabilizes. If you haven't gained back any weight during this time, and if you wish to eat more servings in these categories, by all means do so.

Refer to the Protein Gram Counters that follow (pages 123–130) for the serving sizes and calculate the grams of protein you should be consuming, not to exceed the 50, 60, 75, or 85 grams of protein that apply to you.

Protein Intake Charts

50 Grams per Day Protein Intake

| Food Group | ANTI-AGING DIET SERVINGS PER DAY | |
	Weight Loss	Lifetime Program
1. Fruits and fruit juices	3	Unlimited: meet needs
2. Vegetables Nonstarchy Starchy	 Unlimited 2	 Unlimited Unlimited: meet needs
3. Cereals and grains	2	Unlimited: meet needs
4. Legumes Nuts and seeds	1 or 2, depending on animal protein consumed 1 or 2 per week	Unlimited: use as a substitute for animal protein 2 or 3 times per week 1 or 2 per week
5. Animal products	About 25 grams of protein (for example, 1 serving milk and 2 1-ounce servings of fish, poultry, or meat)	25 grams of protein (for example, 1 serving of milk and 2 1-ounce servings of fish, poultry, or meat)
Flavor Enhancers		
Fats	2	Not more than 3 or 4
Sugars	2	Not more than 3 or 4

60 Grams per Day Protein Intake

Food Group	ANTI-AGING DIET SERVINGS PER DAY	
	Weight Loss	*Lifetime Program*
1. Fruit	4	Unlimited: meet needs

2. Vegetables
   Nonstarchy
   Starchy
	Unlimited
	2
		Unlimited
		Unlimited: meet needs

3. Cereals and grains	2	Unlimited: meet needs
4. Legumes Nuts and seeds	1 or 2, depending on animal protein consumed 1 or 2 per week	Unlimited: use as a substitute for animal protein 2 or 3 times per week 1 or 2 per week
5. Animal products	About 30 grams of protein (for example, 1 serving milk and 3 1-ounce servings of fish, poultry, or meat)	About 30 grams of protein (for example, 1 serving milk and 3 1-ounce servings of fish, poultry, or meat)
Flavor Enhancers		
Fats Sugars	2 2	Not more than 3 or 4 Not more than 3 or 4

75 Grams per Day Protein Intake

Food Group	ANTI-AGING DIET SERVINGS PER DAY	
	Weight Loss	Lifetime Program
1. Fruit	5	Unlimited: meet needs

2. Vegetables
  Nonstarchy
  Starchy
	Unlimited
	3
		Unlimited
		Unlimited: meet needs

3. Cereals and grains	3	Unlimited: meet needs
4. Legumes Nuts and seeds	1 or 2, depending on animal protein consumed 1 or 2 per week	Unlimited within protein requirements: use as a substitute for animal protein 2 or 3 times per week 1 or 2 per week
5. Animal products	About 38 grams of protein (for example, 1 serving milk and 4 1-ounce servings fish, poultry, or meat)	About 38 grams of protein (for example, 1 serving milk and 4 1-ounce servings fish, poultry, or meat)
Flavor Enhancers		
Fats	3	Not more than 3 or 4
Sugars	2	Not more than 3 or 4

85 Grams per Day Protein Intake

| Food Group | ANTI-AGING DIET SERVINGS PER DAY | |
	Weight Loss	Lifetime Program
1. Fruit	6	Unlimited: meet needs

2. Vegetable
   Nonstarchy
   Starchy
	Unlimited
	3
		Unlimited
		Unlimited: meet needs

3. Grains	4	Unlimited: meet needs
4. Legumes Nuts and seeds	1 or 2, depending on animal protein consumed 2 or 3 per week	Unlimited within protein requirements: use as a substitute for animal protein 2 or 3 times per week 2 or 3 per week
5. Animal products	About 42 grams of protein (for example, 2 servings milk and 4 1-ounce servings fish, poultry, or meat)	About 42 grams of protein (for example, 2 servings milk and 4 1-ounce servings fish, poultry, or meat)
Flavor Enhancers		
Fats Sugars	3 2	Not more than 3 or 4 Not more than 3 or 4

Protein-Gram Counters

FOOD GROUP 1: FRUITS AND FRUIT JUICES

Any whole, fresh fruit is recommended; this partial listing will give you an idea of appropriate serving sizes. Avoid fruits and juices with added sugar.

FOOD	GRAMS OF PROTEIN PER SERVING	AVERAGE SERVING SIZE
Apple, pear, peach	Protein is minimal in this food group. Count all fruits as having 0 grams of protein	4 ounces
Banana		½
Berries, all kinds		1 cup
Dates, dried		2
Grape juice		¼ cup
Grapes		About 20
Mango		4 ounces
Melon		1 cup
Orange juice		½ cup
Orange or grapefruit		About 5 ounces
Papaya		1 cup
Pineapple		1 cup
Prune juice		¼ cup
Prunes		4
Raisins		2 tablespoons

FOOD GROUP 2: VEGETABLES
NONSTARCHY VEGETABLES AND VEGETABLE JUICES

A serving is 1 cup of raw or ½ cup cooked vegetables.

FOOD	GRAMS OF PROTEIN PER SERVING
Asparagus Bean sprouts Beets Broccoli Brussels sprouts Carrots Cauliflower Celery Cucumbers Eggplant Greens (leafy, all varieties): beet, chard, collard, kale, spinach, turnip, watercress Jicama Lettuce, all varieties Mushrooms Okra Onions Peppers, all varieties Radishes String beans Summer squash Tomatoes Turnips Vegetable juices, unsalted or low salt	Count as 2 grams of protein per serving

STARCHY VEGETABLES

This group of vegetables contains more carbohydrate than the previous group and provides a valuable source of vegetable protein.

FOOD	GRAMS OF PROTEIN PER SERVING	AVERAGE SERVING SIZE
Corn	3	½ cup
Potato, white	3	5 ounces
Potato, sweet/yam,	2	½ cup
Popcorn, air-popped	3	4 cups
Pumpkin, cooked	2	1 cup
Squash, acorn, cooked	2	1 cup
Squash, butternut, cooked	2	1 cup
Squash, hubbard, cooked	4	1 cup
Squash, spaghetti, cooked	1	1 cup
Succotash	5	½ cup

FOOD GROUP 3: CEREALS AND GRAINS

This group includes products made from the cereal grains—barley, corn, rice, oats, wheat, rye, and millet.

FOOD	GRAMS OF PROTEIN PER SERVING	AVERAGE SERVING SIZE
Bagel	2	1 ounce or ½
Barley, cooked	3	⅓ cup
Breads, whole grain	2–4	1 ounce
Bulgur, cooked	4	½ cup
Cereals, ready to eat	1–6	½ to 1 cup (read labels and choose cereals not sugar-coated, with 4 to 10 grams of dietary fiber per serving)
Cornmeal, white or yellow, dry	2	3 tablespoons
Corn tortilla	2	1 ounce
Cream of wheat, cooked	3	¾ cup
Flour (wheat) tortilla	3	1 ounce
Oat bran, hot cereal, cooked	6	¾ cup
Oatmeal, cooked	5	¾ cup
Pasta, cooked	2–4	½ cup
Pancake	2	1 ounce
Pita pocket	4	1½ ounces
Rice, brown or white, cooked	2	½ cup
Wheat bran, dry	2	2 tablespoons
Wheat germ, toasted	0.4	1 tablespoon
Wheatena	4	¾ cup

FOOD GROUP 4: LEGUMES, NUTS, AND SEEDS

Legumes

Foods in this grouping are rich in protein and should be eaten either in place of animal protein two or three times a week or in combination with small amounts of animal foods.

FOOD	GRAMS OF PROTEIN PER SERVING	AVERAGE SERVING SIZE
Beans, black, cooked	6	½ cup
Beans, garbanzo, cooked	7	½ cup
Beans, kidney, cooked	6	½ cup
Beans, lima, cooked	7	½ cup
Beans, mung, cooked	10	½ cup
Beans, navy, cooked	8	½ cup
Beans, pinto, cooked	7	½ cup
Lentils, cooked	9	½ cup
Peas, black-eyed, cooked	6	½ cup
Peas, green, cooked from frozen	4	½ cup
Peas, split green, cooked	8	½ cup
Tofu (soybean curd)	8	½ cup

Nuts and Seeds

Members of this group are high in calories and you should limit the number of servings you eat to maintain your ideal weight.

FOOD	GRAMS OF PROTEIN PER SERVING	AVERAGE SERVING SIZE
Almonds	4	2 tablespoons
Cashews	2	2 tablespoons
Peanuts, roasted	4	2 tablespoons
Peanut butter	5	1 tablespoon
Pecans	1	2 tablespoons
Pine nuts	3	2 tablespoons
Pumpkin seeds	4	2 tablespoons
Sesame seeds	5	2 tablespoons
Sunflower seeds	4	2 tablespoons
Walnuts	2	2 tablespoons

FOOD GROUP 5: ANIMAL PRODUCTS

Includes all foods that originate with animals such as meat, fish, poultry, eggs, milk, cheese, and yogurt. To keep fat within current health guidelines, choose low-fat animal products when appropriate. Limit the amount of animal protein you eat to half your daily protein intake. The remainder should be from plant foods. Serving sizes for meat, fish, and poultry are gauged after cooking.

FOOD	GRAMS OF PROTEIN PER SERVING	AVERAGE SERVING SIZE
Beef, lean	9	1 ounce
Cheese, low fat	8	1 ounce
Cheese, cottage, lowfat	14	½ cup
Cheese, ricotta, part skim	7	¼ cup
Egg, white	3	1
Egg, whole	6	1
Fish (most varieties)	7	1 ounce
Milk, skim or 1%	8	1 cup
Pork, tenderloin, roasted	9	1 ounce
Poultry, lean	8	1 ounce
Seafood (lobster, scallops, shrimp)	7	1 ounce
Tuna, canned in water	8	1 ounce
Yogurt, nonfat	10–13	1 cup

FLAVOR ENHANCERS: FATS AND SWEETS

Added fats and sugars including artificial sweeteners contain no protein. They are used as flavor enhancers and often add many unnecessary, empty calories. Therefore, they are not considered a food group on the Anti-Aging Diet. Their use should always be *limited* if not eliminated.

Fats

FOOD	GRAMS OF PROTEIN PER SERVING	AVERAGE SERVING SIZE
Vegetable oils	Count all fats as 0 grams protein	1 teaspoon
Olive oil		1 teaspoon
Margarine or butter		1 teaspoon
Regular salad dressings		1 tablespoon
Regular mayonnaise		½ tablespoon

Sugars

FOOD	GRAMS OF PROTEIN PER SERVING	AVERAGE SERVING SIZE
Sugar or honey	Simple sugar contains no protein; count as 0 grams of protein	1 teaspoon
Jam, jelly, or marmalade		1 teaspoon
Apple butter		1 tablespoon

Foods of Animal Origin: Rare to Almost Never Listed

While protein content of these foods may be similar to or even less than that of comparable foods listed on the anti-aging lifetime diet, the following foods are not recommended as a part of your diet because they are so high in fat and/or sodium.

FOOD	GRAMS OF PROTEIN PER SERVING	AVERAGE SERVING SIZE
Bacon	2	1 slice
Bologna	3	1 ounce
Cheese, Cheddar, regular	7	1 ounce
Cheese, cream, regular	2	1 ounce
Cream, half and half	0.4	1 tablespoon
Hamburger	22	3 ounces
Hot dog (beef and pork)	5	1
Ice cream, vanilla	5	1 cup
Liver, calf, fried	30	3½ ounces
Pepperoni	1	1 slice (0.25 ounce)
Pork chops	23	3 ounces
Sausage, pork	9	2-ounce patty
Salami, pork and beef	2	½-ounce slice
Steak, T-bone	24	3 ounces
Sour cream	0.4	1 tablespoon
Spare ribs, pork	29	3 ounces
Whipping cream	0.3	1 tablespoon

All values from *Food Values*, by Pennington and Church, 14th ed.

When eating combination foods such as soup, protein content will be dependent on the types and amounts of foods included.

Chapter 6

Shopping, Cooking, and Eating the Anti-Aging Way

As you begin to assimilate the Anti-Aging Diet into your life, you'll become aware of certain changes affecting your attitudes toward shopping, cooking, socializing over food with friends—and even toward the most basic of physical functions, eliminating.

The process of deciding what to eat, how to eat, and when to eat is an unconscious choice for many, but it's got to become a deliberate conscious choice for you if you intend to change your old habits and live better as you live longer.

Believe me, after you've been with the healthful and easy to follow Anti-Aging Diet for a couple of weeks, you'll hardly recall living any other way. Initially, however, you're going to need a few reminders and a lot of encouragement. Don't worry, it gets incredibly simple very quickly!

Going Shopping the Anti-Aging Way

If you usually spend about an hour in the supermarket doing your shopping for the week, I want you to time yourself to see how long you spend in each section. If you find yourself lingering over the meat and poultry or the dairy aisle, you're in the wrong place for the wrong amount of time!

From now on, I want you to apportion your shopping hour this way:

- *20 minutes* getting vegetables and fruits:
  Be as creative and experimental as you like in the produce section. Remember that you can use vegetables in main dishes and salads, raw or cooked. You'll be eating at least one carrot a day to get the beta carotene you need, so buy a large bag. Fruit can be snacks or desserts or breakfast food, again, eaten raw or cooked.

- *25 minutes* getting cereal, grains, and legumes:
  —In the grains aisle get pasta, rice, cornmeal, wheat berries, barley, kasha.
  —In the bread aisle pick whole grain bread, bagels, and pita.
  —In the cereals aisle choose ready-to-eat cereals that are high in fiber and low in sugar, please; or bran cereals and oatmeal, which are your best choices. Although oat bran cereals are high in fiber and carbohydrates and are therefore beneficial, they will do nothing to reduce your cholesterol level unless you eat massive quantities of them—which would undoubtedly cause abdominal distension and excess gas.
  —In the aisle that has legumes get beans, lentils, dried peas, peanuts, and nuts and seeds, such as sunflower or sesame seeds. Beans and lentils are high in protein; nuts and seeds are high in both protein and fat. And plant protein is much less stressful on your kidneys and liver.

- *15 minutes* for animal protein:
  —In the meat, poultry, and fish aisle you can now get the ingredients for your side dishes. When you get home from the market, you'll have to open your meat packages and cut the meat into individual-meal portions so they can be frozen and used later.
  —In the dairy products aisle get skim milk or 1-percent milk, nonfat yogurt, low-fat cheese, low-fat sour cream or substitute, eggs or egg substitutes.

• And even more briefly, spend a moment or two in the aisle that has monunsaturated and polyunsaturated oils.

EXTRA SHOPPING TIPS

• Always read labels. Be sure to check the fat and sodium content of all products. Food packagers are now required to provide this information. Many dry cereals are very high in sodium and the supposedly "healthy" granola varieties are also high in fat.
• You don't need to buy a cereal that's touted as having "complete RDAs." You'll be eating enough of the recommended daily allowances of all foods with the rest of your diet.
• When you do buy meat, buy only lean varieties, trimmed of fat.
• When you get poultry home, immediately discard the skin—it's much too high in fat. Think of it as something tossed in to make your package weigh and cost more. Remove and discard any visible fat, too.
• Forget about buying soda, which is high in sugar or sugar substitutes, caffeine, and phosphates; buy bottled water, juice, or flavored seltzer instead.
• Remember that yogurt is higher in protein than milk, so if you select it as one of your animal proteins for the day, you may need to cut down your protein allowance at your next meal.

GENERAL HINTS FOR FOOD PREPARATION

- Bake, broil, poach, or steam foods instead of frying them.
- If a recipe calls for eggs, use one egg white for every other whole egg.
- Cook with monounsaturated oils such as peanut or olive oil; or polyunsaturated oils such as soybean, sunflower, safflower, corn, and cottonseed oils; never with the saturated fats— butter, palm, or coconut oil.
- Instead of sautéing or refrying in oil, cook in a little milk or broth.
- Serve salads with Mexican salsa instead of salad dressing— they come in mild, moderate, and hot varieties—or you can make your own (see recipes pages 223 and 224). Salsa is a tomato-based sauce without a lot of heavy oil that spices up a salad without adding a lot of fats or calories.
- If you didn't throw out the poultry skin when you came home from the market, discard it before you start cooking.
- Use garlic, pepper, thyme, dill, coriander, sage, oregano, paprika, and other herbs and spices instead of salt to season food.
- Trim meat of any excess fat before cooking.
- Cook meats, poultry, and fish on racks so that the fats can run off into the pan.

How to Eat Out

Whether you're dining out with friends or having dinner at someone's home, eating out can often be problematic when you're on any kind of diet. Some dieters tend to be fanatics, feeling that any nutritional faux pas will land them right back at square one, with every lost pound gained back. Some dieters are strict at home but forget everything they ever knew about eating when they're in a social situation, rationalizing that they can always "be good again" tomorrow.

I remember I once had a patient who was a senator who needed to lose 30 pounds in six months, by the time his next election rolled around. Carrying around those extra 30 pounds was not only bad for his health and longevity, it was bad for his image, and he was concerned that his constituents wouldn't continue to support him if he didn't look as good as his younger, thinner opponent.

Naturally, like most politicians, he was constantly on the "rubber chicken" circuit. When he started the Anti-Aging Diet, he assured me he would try his best, but what could he do at a cocktail party when he was served alcohol, or at a fundraiser when the main course was tournedos of beef swimming in béarnaise sauce? Also, although he had not made his opposition to broccoli quite as vehement as that of another public figure we know, he was inordinately stubborn about not eating other vegetables.

I told him he could have Perrier or juice instead of a cocktail, that he could eat plenty of bread and potatoes, and even be daring enough to request a plate of pasta for his main course. He actually did lose 20 of his 30 pounds by the next election, and he gave up wine and French cuisine, as well.

He'd gone from 195 to 175 pounds, true, but I don't think he really understood his total clinical picture until I showed him the astounding results. His cholesterol decreased from 380 to 185; his blood pressure dropped from 150/90 on medication to 120/80 without medication. Where six out of ten of his liver function scores had been elevated, now only one was elevated, and his kidney function score had improved from 30 to 18.

Like the senator, you have to realize that no matter what's going on in your life right now, you're eating not just for today but for the future. It doesn't make sense to keep a double standard, behaving in a pristine manner in your own home while you go wild in a restaurant. It also doesn't make any sense to put down your fork and leave the table in a snit because someone has offered you a thick steak and a pitcher of hollandaise to pour on your asparagus.

Let's think about ways we can adhere to our new way of thinking about food while not totally ignoring the rest of the world. You don't have to bring your own salad dressing and rice to a party nor do you have to consume every bit of cream cake that's served.

I believe that maintaining the Anti-Aging Diet shouldn't make you neurotic. You don't have to be compulsive about discovering how much salt was used in preparing your food or the calorie count and amount of cholesterol in every morsel that passes your mouth.

Let preparation be your guide. If you're in a restaurant, look for these words:

- grilled
- steamed
- broiled
- poached

These methods all suggest the food was probably prepared with less fat. If you see the word "fried," keep moving down the page. Avoid fried foods at all costs! Other methods, such as sautéing, definitely use butter. Foods that are baked may have butter added to toppings, so they should probably be avoided, too. Sauces are usually full of butter and salt.

Complying with the Anti-Aging Diet in a restaurant may be easier than you think. Since you're going to be cutting down on animal fat, you can skip the meat and poultry listings and go instead to the appetizers, pastas, and vegetables. When you reduce the amount of protein in your diet, you will necessarily limit your intake of animal fat.

For example, when you order a pizza, ask for it without cheese or pepperoni but with tomato sauce, green peppers, onions, and mushrooms. This pizza contains half the protein and fat of regular pizza.

Order Chinese food that's not deep fried or breaded—stay away from dumplings and egg rolls. Choose dishes that contain fish or chicken as a condiment mixed with the noodles and vegetables, such as chicken lo mein or moo shu. Rice, of course, is absolutely plain and great for you. If you're in a congenial group, order several vegetable and noodle dishes and only one poultry or fish dish. Tofu or soybean, vegetables, and noodles in Chinese cooking are excellent sources of protein and will supply you with ample amounts for your daily requirement.

If you decide on a fast-food restaurant, go straight to the salad bar, which most now provide. Don't pour creamy dressings over your salad; eat it plain or with an oil and vinegar dressing on the side. Dip your fork in the dressing, then into your salad. Many fast-food places now serve wheat bread or crackers at the salad bar.

When eating out, I suggest you be alert to any "nutritional sirens" that may go off in your head and "speed bumps" over which you must slow down. These would be sauces, toppings, and fillings of unknown composition.

Red lights will bring you to a complete stop. These include high-protein foods, high-fat foods, and simple carbohydrates, i.e., refined sugar.

But here are the green lights: fresh vegetables, salads, legumes, fruits, breads, and other complex carbohydrates, especially whole grains.

You don't need to be terribly concerned about the salt content of most restaurant foods unless you suffer from heart disease or high blood pressure. If so, ask to have your food prepared without salt, and do not salt it at the table.

Finally, don't be afraid to ask for exceptions and alterations in the printed menu when you're dining out. It's fairly common knowledge that famous movie stars *never* order what's on the menu but always test the chef by requesting their own version of what they want to eat. This may be either a power trip or a diet trip, or both! When you think about the fact that most restaurants have a wide variety of most edible items back in the kitchen, it becomes easier. "May I have that fish grilled without butter?" is a perfectly acceptable question. "Would you mind serving my baked potato dry, with a little vinegar or salsa on the side?" sounds awfully nice.

You'll be surprised at how accommodating most restaurants— from the fanciest to the least expensive—can be. Anything that's intended to be prepared with a sauce can be made without; anything that's supposed to be broiled in butter can be broiled dry or with lemon juice. And rice is rice. Pasta is pasta. Plain and simple.

Now, what about being invited to a friend's house? It's not exactly polite to ask for something other than what's being served, nor is it gracious to bring a brown bag when you come to an elegant dinner party. My wife, Molly, and I were recently faced with a challenge like this.

Our host was a senator from Arizona, John McCain. Molly was seated between Senator McCain and John Teets, who is chairman of the board of the Greyhound/Dial Corporation. They were having a fine time talking when the meal was served—vegetables, potatoes, and the *pièce de résistance*, a large haunch of veal.

Molly has been a vegetarian for the past four years. She simply avoided the meat and was enjoying the rest of her meal when the senator asked if everything was to her liking. She told him with a smile that the vegetables were very well prepared. What else could she say?

But at this point, I figured that honesty was the better part of valor and, as the residing health and nutrition expert, I thought that no one would mind my putting in my two cents. I said very simply that Molly and I were both vegetarians and would be very happy with more vegetables. Our plates were promptly refilled. Several others at the table volunteered that they would love to become vegetarians but they didn't think they had the will power. They admired us greatly for complying with our diets.

The highlight of the meal was dessert—a large bowl of fresh strawberries—which Molly and I took great pleasure in eating.

It never hurts to be honest. At the very least, you'll get some good conversation going about the merits and demerits of various different nutritional beliefs.

My suggestion, when you're faced with a meal of steak or pork roast at someone's home, is to ask for extra vegetables, extra salad, and additional bread. You can ignore the main course (leaving more for everyone who's not on the Anti-Aging Diet) without appearing ungracious about the rest of the food.

But you may find, after having your friends over and serving them some of the Anti-Aging Diet soups, stews, pastas, and salads, that your friends may so delight in the new flavors and the fantastic way they feel at the end of a meal that they'll be begging you to teach them how to cook in a more nutritionally sound fashion, with less protein and more complex carbohydrates.

What About Spices and Dietary Fiber?

The digestive process of your body consists of many different physiological reactions.

Food that contains a lot of fiber can cause a certain amount of abdominal distension and increased movement through the digestive tract. It takes much less time for a piece of bread to pass through your system than a hot dog. This rapid movement may cause gas pressure, cramping, and flatulence, particularly when you're first switching over from a high- to a low-protein diet.

The high-fiber quotient of the Anti-Aging Diet—the peas, beans, and cruciferous vegetables like cabbage, Brussels sprouts, and cauliflower—means that intestinal gas may become a frequent companion, at least while your body adapts to getting a larger proportion of these foods. Other foods that commonly produce gas are raw carrots, celery, eggplant, onions, bananas, apples, raisins, grapes, oat bran and other bran cereals, and for some, milk and milk products. What used to be called roughage foods give you plenty of dietary fiber and so are enormously beneficial. A study done in Finland several years ago showed that people who fasted on cabbage juice for one week—very high in fiber—had a complete resolution of their stomach ulcers.

You will also note that most of the anti-aging recipes call for lots of spices. Not too long ago it was thought that highly spiced foods upset the stomach and that as people aged they should concentrate on blander foods. Not so!

Think if you will about the curries of India and the fiery peppers and chilis consumed by young and old in such diverse regions as Indonesia, China, Thailand, Mexico, and our own American Southwest. No one tones down the spiciness of foods in any of these countries as they age. As a matter of fact, we see less incidence of colon cancer, ulcers, diverticulosis, and gastritis in all of these regions and countries.

Getting Used to Eating Differently

The renewal process of your body may take several months, during which time you may notice a certain amount of abdominal distress. You may say, "I didn't feel so bad before I began this diet, and now I'm having symptoms I never had before." That's simply because you haven't yet realized what feeling really good means. And as your body adjusts, as it inevitably will, you will discover that your digestive system is functioning much better than it ever has. If you are not currently a high-fiber eater, I want you to get yourself onto fiber slowly and gradually in order to allow your body time to get used to a new digestive process. Select fewer servings of high-fiber foods at the beginning of your program, and add one a week.

If you do experience excessive bloating, flatulence, indigestion, abdominal distension, diarrhea and/or constipation, you may want to try adding Lactase to your milk or drinking Lactaid, which is easier for many people to digest. There is also a product on the market called Beano, available at most pharmacies, that contains an enzyme that assists the stomach in breaking down certain foods. A few drops can be sprinkled on gas-producing vegetables—the taste is similar to that of soy sauce. It's helpful to drink lots of water as you become used to eating differently. Pumping at least eight glasses of water through your system is an additional aid to making the food you consume easier to pass, and it's called for on the diet.

In general, I advise you not to worry about these minor discomforts. They simply represent a rite of passage on the road to good health and longer life, necessary but cleansing.

Chapter 7

Exercise: Less Pain, More Sane

I've already told you that there are no magic pills to make you younger, thinner, stronger, faster, or happier. But maybe I was wrong. There is one drug I want you to take when you're on the Anti-Aging Diet, and you have to take it every day for it to be effective. That drug is exercise.

If this seems like a strange concept to you, bear with me for a minute. When I first began working on my concept of the Anti-Aging Diet, it was with the sole intention of making my body a more efficient machine that would stand up over the years without any need for major repairs. I was already hooked on exercise and knew from my reading that the right foods would enhance my potential as a runner.

But in my medical practice, I had to work backwards. I had to take inveterate couch potatoes and drag them kicking and screaming out of doors or into a gym. I had to show them how the low-protein life-style only works when you combine it with daily aerobic movement. And the amazing thing was that people who had never taken the time to walk, swim, jog, bike, or take a dance class kept coming back with reports that they actually enjoyed what they were doing.

Dan, a 38-year-old executive who'd lived with stress and high blood pressure and about 30 extra pounds all his adult life, came to me after four weeks on the Anti-Aging Diet and said, "I can't believe how much I'm getting out of the exercise part of the program. Somehow, doing it makes me want to do more. And doing more makes me feel even better about what I'm eating. And what I'm eating makes me energetic enough to go out and run around again."

Why did this happen to Dan? Because I gave him a drug and he became addicted to it. A healthy addiction, but he couldn't live without it. His body and mind changed together in their orientation toward fitness, until he found that by implementing an exercise plan he would make his diet work even better for him.

Exercise Every Day

A fifteen- or twenty-minute walk, or swim, or jog, or workout of any sort once a day, every day, keeps the doctor away and will keep you young and strong to your hundredth birthday and beyond. I'm not talking about going for the burn, running yourself into the ground or pumping iron until your muscles are screaming for mercy. A brisk walk is great! But you must take a walk a day.

Unlike most experts who recommend a longer period of exercise four or five times a week, I'm telling you to do less, but do it more often. Without fail, it's got to be *every day* on the Anti-Aging Diet program.

Don't exhaust yourself! A minimum of exercise keeps you fit.

The Cooper Clinic Institute for Aerobics Research in Dallas, Texas, found that by walking just two miles a day in 30 to 40 minutes, you can achieve a moderate level of fitness that can make a huge difference in the way you feel and in the way your body responds. As a matter of fact, a recent study of 3,600 moderate exercisers indicates that those who walked four and a half hours a week were half as likely to have elevated cholesterol levels as those who only walked half an hour to two hours a week.[1]

Why is exercise so absolutely essential to maintaining health and preventing illness—perhaps even to extending your life?

Exercise:

- burns calories, allowing you to eat more
- lowers your risk of heart disease and certain cancers
- makes you feel so good about yourself that you become more aware of what and how much you eat
- lowers your stress level
- improves your blood sugar level
- improves your lung capacity
- improves cardiovascular function
- increases muscle strength
- lowers cholesterol levels
- keeps your bones strong and your joints flexible
- improves balance, thereby preventing falls and other injuries
- prevents constipation
- improves your sleep patterns
- decreases depression and fatigue
- improves your ability to think and remember
- improves your appearance—gives you a "glow"
- keeps you biologically younger than your chronological age

And as if all the above reasons weren't enough, exercise has been shown to make a marked difference in the overall quality of life—when you feel better about yourself physically, you tend to make changes that lead to feeling better in general. If modern science were ever to invent a magic pill to put into the body to improve your overall sense of well-being, it couldn't have any greater impact than exercise.

How Fit Do You Have to Be to Live Longer?

A Stanford University School of Medicine study of 17,000 Harvard alumni found that those who burned more than 2,000 calories a week during exercising had a death rate from all causes that was

28 percent lower than that of less active men. This landmark study showed that the risk of death became progressively lower as physical activity level increased from 500 to 3,500 calories burned per week.

Three miles of walking or running a day will burn those 2,000 calories and help you to live not just longer but better. The actual extension of your life span isn't that much—the most recent longevity studies have shown that daily exercise will only add on one to two additional years.

However, the chief benefit of being physically fit is that you'll feel better now and as long as you're alive. And most importantly, you'll be able to keep yourself out of long-term care and continue to function independently no matter what advanced age you achieve. You'll spend less money on doctor visits, need fewer medications, and have all the energy in the world to go out and start a new business, meet a new mate, or travel around the world. According to findings at the Dallas Cooper Clinic,[2] physical fitness makes a difference by protecting you from life-threatening disease:

- Cancer death rates were lower with higher levels of physical fitness
- High fitness ratings were beneficial even to those people with other risk factors, like high blood pressure, elevated cholesterol levels, smoking, and a family history of heart disease

Getting Younger by Feeling More Energized

When a patient comes into my office complaining of fatigue and a variety of physical symptoms that have no apparent physical cause, I always prescribe a daily walk. Inevitably, the symptoms improve or even vanish.

Jack and Phoebe, a couple in their late thirties, came to me because both of them were exhausted all the time. They suspected chronic fatigue syndrome. I ran them through a battery of laboratory tests and discovered that they were in fine shape medically, but when I did a case history on them and found out that neither of them even so much as walked to the corner to get a newspaper, I prescribed my first-line medication, exercise.

Within three weeks of walking together every morning, they both rallied. Though neither of them had believed me when I told them their anxiety and depression would lessen on the anti-aging plan, in fact, they commented that a variety of other ailments—insomnia, gastric distress, lower back pain—had somehow resolved themselves over this time period. Each one commented to me separately that they "felt like a kid again." They were laughing more, complaining less. What was going on here? Their commitment to physical activity had mediated both mind and body functions.

What causes the lessening in anxiety and depression associated with exercise? Is it physical, biochemical, or just an emotional response to doing something that's good for you?

Compounds in the brain known as beta endorphins, which are similar in structure to opiates, have been linked to this positive response. Studies suggest that people who exercise for 15 minutes or more daily raise their beta endorphin levels. This rise produces an effect very much like addiction—although, of course, it's a healthy addiction.

The more you do, the more you feel you can do. This is an emotional as well as a physical response. And it is the response typical of a younger person who feels that the world is filled with opportunities that must be taken. As exercise makes your body feel better, you start to see everything in a more positive light.

Why Just a Little Exercise Is Better

I only want you to exercise a little. This is a very powerful drug and I don't want any overdoses. I'm still assuming you'll get hooked, but you shouldn't overdo, even then. The important thing is to get yourself onto the program gradually and build up your tolerance and ability slowly, at your own pace. Too many would-be exercisers have been totally discouraged by difficult or impossible programs that have you running like a rat on a treadmill. If you do too much, too soon, you may injure yourself or simply get so frustrated with your initially low fitness level that you stop altogether.

Most people think exercise must be painful to be beneficial. Just the opposite is true. I only want you to elevate your heart rate to 130 beats a minute or less depending on your age. Here's the formula you follow:

Subtract your age from 220, then take 70 percent of that. Your heart rate should never exceed this number when you're exercising.

Sweating has nothing to do with losing weight, nor do aches and pains mean you're really disciplined. If you stretch properly before you begin, you reduce the risk of injury and, what's most important, you eliminate the possibility of giving up your exercise program entirely because you're so frustrated at your lack of stamina and ability. Exercise for the '90s works on the principle *less pain, more sane.*

When starting an exercise program you must also:

- get your physician's okay
- wear appropriate shoes and clothing
- replenish lost liquids by drinking plenty of water
- warm up before you begin

The best thing about exercise is that there's such diversity and so many forms of activity that complement each other. The more you do, the more you'll want to do.

WHEN TO EXERCISE

It's been found that compliance with an exercise program is far likelier for most people first thing, as soon as they wake up, even with those who don't consider themselves "morning people." Just by setting the alarm a few minutes earlier, you can do some stretching, get in a brisk walk, jog, or swim, then take your shower and get ready for the day.

Those who begin an exercise program at some other time of day are more likely to slack off or drop out. It's harder to accommodate the extra time in your schedule for a midday exercise session, and it's easy to come up with excuses when you're locked into an evening session. Also, people are tired after a full day of work and/or child care, and they just don't feel like putting on sweats and fitting in their workout.

Daily Exercise Is the Only Way to Lose Weight

My patients are the best proof that there is no anti-aging success without exercise and that exercise accelerates both the diet and the anti-aging process.

I noticed that the patients who were losing weight very slowly would confess, after a little prodding, that they just didn't have the time or energy to take that fifteen-minute walk a day. The patients who lost weight quickly (even those who had been classified as obese when they first came to see me) were those who complied completely with the daily exercise regime I gave them.

Alice, who was 36—a stunning woman—was one hundred pounds overweight when she came to the Southwest Health Institute to see me. Her husband was ridiculously jealous about her looks and had, in a subtle but deliberate manner, encouraged her to eat a lot and stay sedentary after they married so that no other man would ever find his wife sexually attractive. Alice was miserable at our first appointment. She was short of breath and too embarrassed to be seen in public. But she was motivated to get out of her unfortunate situation, so she started on the diet. She listened to my explanation of addictive exercise, but I could tell I wasn't getting through to her.

For the first two months, Alice was diligent about switching to low-protein eating, but told me it was too difficult to exercise. She'd bought an expensive exercise bike, but she was nervous about toppling off it because she felt so unbalanced. She was losing a little weight but not a significant amount.

I told her the diet wasn't going to make a real difference in her life and longevity unless she got out of the house and started moving. I didn't care when she did it—she could go in the middle of the night for all I cared. But she had to walk!

As it happened, my urging came at a time when her husband was away on a long business trip. Alice did, in fact, wake up at 4:00 A.M. each morning for the three weeks that he was gone. And when she came back to me, she proclaimed that the weight was falling off her. And that she actually liked walking! She didn't care what her husband said—she was going to continue.

Nine months and ninety pounds later, Alice was in fantastic shape. She was running three miles a day and swimming three times a week. The personal, emotional, and biochemical changes in this young woman were astounding. She told me that she had never in her life enjoyed each day so much, and she had actually convinced her husband to join her on the anti-aging lifetime program. She also told me that the less protein she ate each week, the more energy she seemed to have for exercise. Of course, this phenomenon is scientifically verifiable. By eating more carbohydrates and less protein, she had supplied her body with just the right fuel for the job it needed to do.

The Interplay Between Diet and Exercise

In 1980, the American Dietetic Association published a statement on the importance of a high-carbohydrate, low-protein diet for the endurance performance of athletes.[3] At that time, they recommended that complex carbohydrates as 60 to 70 percent of daily caloric intake would give the best results.

And it's not only athletes who benefit from a high-carbohydrate, low-protein diet. You don't have to be running marathons or competing in the Olympics to be able to make your body function like a lean, well-tuned machine.

You may recall from Chapter 2 that a doctor named Chittenden at the turn of the century drastically reduced the protein in athletes' diets and greatly improved their performance.

Then, in 1939, Christensen and Hansen firmly established the relationship between a high-carbohydrate diet and the ability of athletes to improve their endurance.[4] They asked three groups of subjects to eat three different diets for three to four days. One was on a normal mixed diet, one ate primarily fat and protein, and the third ate a low-protein diet high in complex carbohydrates. The difference in endurance performance was startling. The endurance capacity almost doubled for those on the low-protein, high-carbohydrate diet.

Recently, researchers in the sports medicine field have done extensive experimentation in moderately active populations as well as in elite athletes such as weight lifters and speed skaters, runners, and cyclists. All the experiments indicated that a comparison of diets high in protein, sucrose, and starch yields conclusive proof that low-protein is the most sparing on the body. There is less nitrogen depletion and better muscle function as well as efficient use of muscle glycogen stores.[5]

Remember what I said earlier about the way the body processes its macronutrients? First it uses its carbohydrate stores, then fat, and then protein for the energy it needs. And the muscle cells—which are activated during any form of exercise—function much more efficiently and give you a better burst of power when they can use their limited glycogen stores in an economical fashion.

A low-protein, high-carbohydrate diet does just this. Your endurance for activity is dependent on how capable your muscles are of tapping into their energy needs. Instead of wasting metabolic energy on digesting protein, the body is immediately getting fuel for exercising from more easily digested carbohydrates. What you eat and what you do in terms of activity dovetail perfectly to make your body more capable, more vital and alive than it's ever been.

Exercise increases the production of enzymes that facilitate energy expenditure and also enlarges the muscle cells of the body so that as your metabolism rate increases, more food is converted more quickly to fuel. The result is that your percentage of lean body tissue goes up and the percentage of fat goes down. The change in proportion of lean muscle mass to fat is the reason why your clothes fit you better even if you haven't lost a pound in a week or so.

Other Benefits of a Daily Exercise Program

There are a variety of other invaluable profits you'll reap from exercising daily:

- Motivation. The more you do, the more you realize you can do. Having lost five pounds and walked two miles, you'll discover you really enjoy the feeling of being lighter and fitter.
- Exercise tones down your appetite. After you've just walked or taken a swim, you'll find you have less desire to eat.
- Exercise makes you burn calories at a higher rate *after* activity. That's right! Exercise increases your metabolic rate and keeps it at this higher rate for six to eight hours after you stop exercising. What this means is that your body continues the process of burning calories that went on during exercise. So even while you're sitting at your desk three hours after your walk, you're burning more calories than on a day you don't exercise.

• Increased capability. As you lose pounds on the Anti-Aging Diet, you'll find it easier to exercise because you're not hauling around so much weight. If a 180-pound man drops to 150, he doesn't burn as many calories in covering his miles—the less you weigh, the less energy you expend covering distance or lifting your body up a flight of stairs.

• Increased energy. Most diets deplete your energy because the foods that usually "keep you going" are forbidden and you feel weak from the sudden loss of daily caloric intake. On the Anti-Aging Diet, however, you're never fatigued because the complex carbohydrates and fiber you're getting are more readily available to the body as energy than protein is. As you exercise, you're immediately putting to use the nutrients in your system and eliminating unnecessary fats or harmful toxins.

You've *got* to put in your fifteen minutes a day! I don't care how you manage it—just *do it!* The only way your new eating plan is going to work for you is if you implement the exercise component along with it. Believe me when I tell you that they are inseparable partners on the road to good health and slowing down the aging process. Proper diet can't exist without exercise, nor will exercise do you any good without a proper diet. It is a sine qua non, which roughly translated from the Latin means "This cannot exist without that."

Creating Your Personal Exercise Program

I remember one of my patients telling me that she just couldn't bring herself to buy a pair of walking shoes. When I asked why, she said it was because she associated exercise with her much-hated gym periods in high school, when she was forced to wear an exceptionally unfashionable gymsuit and attempt to climb a rope attached to the gym ceiling.

Most people who say they hate exercise were introduced to it the wrong way, by a rabid gym teacher or military sergeant barking orders. The calisthenics most of us were forced to perform at an early age were badly taught with little preparation or proper stretching beforehand. And, worse, the exercises just weren't fun or satisfying to do.

I want you to forget everything you ever thought about exercise as a humiliating, time-wasting, difficult activity you got nothing out of. What you're going to imagine now is a life-style change that will promote your good health and your longevity.

There are dozens of good fitness books around to help you in customizing your program. You should first select a form of aerobic exercise—that is, one that gets you huffing and puffing, raises your heart rate, expands your lungs, and usually makes you perspire. Fast walking, jogging, biking, racquet sports, cross country skiing, and strenuous dancing are all forms of aerobics. Swimming is aerobic, and although it's not a weight-bearing exercise since your body is supported by the water, it is a terrific way to keep fit.

And to add variety you can pick an anaerobic exercise a couple of days a week. This type of activity causes your pulse rate to become elevated but does not allow you to maintain that elevated pulse for a sustained period of time. For example, running a hundred-meter dash is an anaerobic form of exercise. It won't burn more calories than a good, slow fifteen-minute jog, though it can increase your cardiovascular benefits. Weight training and isometrics are also forms of anaerobic exercise. They can fit nicely into your fitness program as a complement to the complete, sustained workout you get from aerobic exercise.

You can also select a toning exercise, such as tai ch'i or yoga or any one from the whole family of martial arts—karate, tai kwon do, aikido, kendo—as well as gymnastics, or weight lifting.

Your goal is to have a body and mind that are completely conditioned. For a sound cardiovascular system and a set of lungs that just won't quit, get into walking. For a beautifully toned body, with all the curves in all the right places, lift weights. And for a calmer mind, do tai ch'i or yoga.

The Anti-Aging Option Plan

You can and should mix and match your exercise, depending on your likes, dislikes, and the availability of certain activities. You'll probably find a few options that are just right for you. That's wonderful! If you love to ski and it's summertime, there are a lot of good indoor cross-country ski machines on the market. Also, you can switch to roller-skating or roller-blading until the snow falls again. If you've become a dedicated walker—as most of my patients are—don't worry about the weather. If it's beautiful out, you can go and admire the scenery; if it's miserable out, you can drive to the mall and spend your exercise time doing a brisk few miles there. Mall-walker clubs are springing up all over America.

Once you get used to fitting that activity period into your day, you'll be hooked and will hardly remember a time when you didn't exercise.

You'll be selecting your activities based on factors such as whether you live in a cold or warm climate, whether you like to exercise alone or with a group, whether you like competitive or noncompetitive sports, whether you like to sweat or can't stand sweating, whether you want a longer, slower period of exercise or a shorter, more demanding period. You may decide you want to tone your muscles and tendons, to limber up the mind as well as the body with meditative exercise, or that you want to be as aerobically active as possible.

But whatever you decide, *do it every day!* If you're currently in an exercise program, say an hour-long aerobics class three times a week, that's wonderful! Stick with it. But you must also fit in fifteen minutes on the other days when you don't have class.

If you make the time to shave or put on makeup every day, you can make the time to exercise!

What Does It Mean to Be Fit?

I'm not trying to turn you into a world-class athlete. If it happens (as it has with quite a few of my patients), wonderful. But what we're really looking for in the interest of ongoing good health and longevity is *fitness.*

Fitness means that the body is toned, flexible, and strong. A partial determinant of how fit you are is genetic, but behavior is at least as important, particularly as you age. When you pass 35, your bones lose their density and become more fragile; your muscles tend to sag and weaken, the tendons that cushion the bones become less flexible, if—and that's a big if—you don't exercise.

But if you keep yourself moving every day, you can turn back the chronological clock. Probably everyone's greatest fear about growing older is being unable to care for themselves, that you'll simply hang on, dependent on a younger relative or a long-term care facility. This will never happen to you if you keep yourself vital, strong, and well conditioned.

Just getting up out of that chair and doing something that elevates your pulse consistently lowers your risk of contracting heart disease. It makes your bones strong enough to take you out of the high-risk group for osteoporosis. It lowers your blood pressure, lowers your stress level, and reapportions your body weight so that you look better as well as feel better.

FITNESS TIPS

Here are a few easy changes you can make in your life that will make you more fit:

- Don't take the elevator; climb the stairs
- Walk to the corner store or bus stop; don't drive
- Do isometric exercises for your abdominal muscles while driving the car
- Throw away your remote control. If you're going to watch TV, get up and walk over to it to change the channel; then don't sit but stretch while watching a program

---

If you start thinking about exercise in a new way—not as a grueling form of punishment, but as a positively addictive drug that makes you feel stronger, fitter, less stressed out, and better motivated to stick with your diet—you'll find it not just painless but priceless.

So put down the book, put on your walking shoes, go outside and get started! There's plenty of time to get to the next chapter, *after* you've finished your daily exercise.

Chapter 8

Supplementing Your Low-Protein Diet

Fifteen years ago, I would no more have prescribed vitamins for my patients than I would have prescribed tranquilizers for stress. But as I began to see the amazing benefits of the low-protein life-style, I wanted to know more about exactly what was going on inside the body. As various biochemical changes took place in my patients, and they became healthier because of what they were eating, I saw that they could reach an even higher plateau if they increased the vitamins and minerals they were getting on a dietary basis with supplements.

Today, I recommend that every patient at the Southwest Health Institute supplement the Anti-Aging Diet with the *requisite* vitamins and minerals described at the end of this chapter. Keep reading, to understand just how supplementation enhances weight loss and longevity.

Just a Few Vitamins a Day
Keep the Body Okay

Why take supplements? If you're following the Anti-Aging Diet, shouldn't that give you everything you need? Not really.

We used to think that vitamin pills served to make up for the lack of nutrients in deficient diets—children needed them because of the requirements in each stage of their physical development; pregnant women needed them because of their bodies' increased demand for growth; sick people needed them because their bodies were called upon to do a great deal of extra repair work—all of these cases necessitated more than a regular diet would provide. Vitamins were also for health food nuts who truly believed that processed American foods, sprayed with pesticides and loaded with additives, would kill them otherwise.

But we know today that this is not the case. A regular, balanced diet does not always meet everyone's nutritional needs. A diet low in protein specifically tones and preserves the body's organs so that they can function better for longer periods of time. But in recent years an enormous amount of scientific research has indicated that certain vitamins, minerals, and trace elements—over and above the dietary amounts you take in—are essential in protecting the body from disease and perhaps from the aging process itself.

They can act as carcinogen scavengers, roaming the body and destroying elements that could potentially turn to toxins. And they can also retain the integrity of cell membranes often broken down by the oxidative action of free radicals. The architectural stability of each cell is vital to the healthy performance of the body.

When you have proper supplementation, you are actively working to store up reserves that will protect your body from the natural breakdown process that goes on in your tissues over the years—regardless of what we eat.

Recent studies suggest that the supplements I'm about to recommend prevent heart disease, certain cancers, macular degeneration of the retina, and cataracts and even strengthen the immune system. Just thirty to sixty days after beginning a minimal vitamin and mineral regimen, you will feel better as every system in your body develops a new, impervious barrier against illness.

My Personal Supplement Regimen

As I've explained in earlier chapters, the Anti-Aging Diet has been my best personal proof of the way in which I've grown younger over the last fifteen years. But when I reached a plateau in my running and wasn't progressing at all three years ago, I decided to try supplementation, having read phenomenal reports of the effects of vitamin C and selenium in particular on athletes' improved ability.

For the past three years, I have been taking a multiple vitamin and mineral supplement as well as 400 IUs of vitamin E and 200 micrograms of selenium. This regimen has had a dramatic effect on my physical activity level. When I first began this supplementation, my 10-kilometer (6.2-mile) minimarathon time was forty-eight minutes. Now, it's dropped to forty-two minutes—nearly a minute a mile less, with no additional training.

Good runners typically reach a point in their forties at which they can stabilize their performance level and know they can count on good sustaining power over time. But when supplementing an excellent diet, they can go much further. I have no doubts that the fact that I'm getting faster as I get older is dependent in great part on the vitamins and minerals I take daily. By consuming antioxidants, I'm foiling nature's ability to age me "naturally."

Vitamins and Minerals as Antioxidants

Current research indicates that vitamins and trace minerals will act, in part, as the superheros of twenty-first-century medicine, capable of leaping most diseases in a single bound, faster than a speeding cancer cell, and more powerful than cholesterol-blocking plaque.

Vitamins and minerals are capable of vanquishing the most dastardly cells that threaten our health on a daily basis. They may never cure a particular condition, but they will buoy up the body's ability to fight disease and to recover quickly from any illness it does contract.

Before I begin to elaborate on the values of the various vitamins and trace minerals on the Anti-Aging Diet, you should know something about the chemical reactions in the body that seem to invite disease and trigger the aging process.

The Damage Done by Oxygen: Cross Linking and Free Radicals

Think for a moment about the smooth, soft surface of a baby's skin and the flexible movements of his body. One of the most important elements in the skin is collagen, an important protein that's in all the connective tissue in the body. Now, in your mind, project that baby forward about seventy years—his skin is lined and wrinkled, with very little elasticity in it, his joints have hardened with arthritis. These changes are the result of an inevitable process of aging known as cross linking.

A chemical bond, like a bridge, forms between protein molecules over time. During this chemical reaction a hydrogen bond is formed that also releases an extra ion—a wild chemical reactant known as a free radical—which has nowhere to go. When a cell loses hydrogen that is replaced by oxygen, you have a process known as oxidation. When food spoils, for example, it's because oxidation has occurred.

Free radicals aid and abet the damage that oxygen does in our environment. If you think oxygen is a benign gas, think about a fire raging out of control; think about the metal rusting underneath your car. Both are examples of oxidation. Free radicals cause a breakdown of tissue in the human body just as they allow butter to turn rancid and rubber to harden when exposed to the air. And they react with one another to set off chain reactions that can cause more disruption. Oxidative damage has been linked to the development of such degenerative diseases as cancer, heart disease, cataracts, and arthritis.

Slowing the Aging Process with Antioxidants

Free radicals are most closely linked with the damage theory of aging. As they attack cellular membranes, they start a chain reaction that breaks down the collagen. The protein bridges they form restrict the molecules they bind, making the molecules increasingly rigid and inflexible.

Free radical reactions aren't all bad—they take place all the time as part of normal metabolic processes. But they can easily get out of control—for example, when they attack the body's DNA and cause abnormal growth of cancer cells; or when they degrade the inside of arterial walls or dry up the mucus that works as a lubricant in your joints, or cause pigment to accumulate in the skin—creating those brown "liver" spots most older people develop. There are chemical reactions going on in your body all the time—in response to sunlight, stress, and the foods you eat.

Our body has its own fail-safe mechanism that keeps the free radicals under control: we manufacture many enzymes that combine free radicals with one another, stabilizing and neutralizing them. But ingestion of antioxidants on a daily basis cuts to a minimum the damage that will be done over time to our vital organs. We can supplement our own natural production of these antioxidants and slow the aging process by taking additional doses orally— the major ones are vitamins E and C, the trace mineral selenium, and beta carotene, a precusor of vitamin A that enhances the color of carrots.

The best course of action, however, is to keep dietary protein down. Ingesting more protein than your body needs provides all the more opportunity for cross linkage.

Supplementation for Disease Prevention and Anti-Aging

Certain vitamins and trace minerals can take free radicals and bond them in a process similar to wrapping them up and throwing them away. They can help to strengthen a cell wall and provide it with an impervious shield so free radicals can't penetrate it. These vitamins and trace minerals stop the oxidation process.

Since rust never sleeps and oxygen depletes us over the years of our youthful glow, we must do something to counteract the damaging effects of free radicals in the body if we intend to increase our maximum life span effectively. Vitamins and minerals are not substitutes for anything; you can't make up for terrible eating habits, lack of exercise, a couple of packs of cigarettes, and a six-pack of beer a day. Rather, vitamins are supplements that must be used in conjunction with the Anti-Aging Diet and always with the approval of your physician.

How Much Will a Vitamin Regimen Cost?

The money you are now pouring into blood pressure– or cholesterol-lowering medication, into antidepressants or tranquilizers will go a long way at the vitamin store. You will probably have to shop around to find the best bargains, but in most parts of the country, you can buy yourself a lot of health for only $10 a month. The cumulative effect of taking vitamins over time is like the "invisible protective shield" they used to advertise with toothpaste—you don't know it's there, but it's working all the time.

The Golden Ones: C, E, Selenium, Calcium, and Beta Carotene

VITAMIN C

I've noticed that people who pooh-pooh vitamin regimens always and unfailingly drink more orange juice when they're getting a cold. The reason, I suspect, is the excellent work done by Dr. Linus Pauling in touting megadoses of ascorbic acid as the cure for the common cold.

But let me tell you about vitamin C's antioxidant virtues, which make it even more valuable than the Nobel laureate imagined when he first popularized his theory back in the 1970s. It would be wonderful to eliminate colds, of course, but perhaps even more useful to understand the mechanisms vitamin C employs in the prevention and treatment of so many degenerative diseases and other conditions. It's been shown to:

- prevent cancer and heart disease
- fight infection
- help heal wounds and speed recovery from surgery
- help prevent blood clots
- help control allergies
- protect the lens of the eye from cataract formation
- assist in collagen synthesis

Good food sources of vitamin C are broccoli, oranges, and papaya.

Drs. Gey, Brubacher, and Stahelin reported[1] recently that incidence of cardiovascular disease and cancer were lower in populations in which individuals consumed plenty of green leafy vegetables and fruit—both of which contain lots of ascorbic acid. And the incidence of both ischemic heart disease and cancer was lower as the dietary level of vitamin C increased.

Vitamin C, which is water soluble, can permeate every cell of the body except fat cells, which is one reason it's so useful in disease prevention.

VITAMIN E

This vitamin is truly amazing. Also known as DI-alpha tocopherol acetate, it is fat soluble and therefore can do its antioxidant work in fatty tissues, where water-soluble vitamin C cannot go. Because oxidation occurs when fat molecules in our cell membranes are involved in free-radical reactions, vitamin E is particularly vital in slowing the aging process in the tissues of the brain, heart, liver, and spinal column.

Vitamin E acts to stabilize the cell membranes and prevent their breakdown. For this reason, it can:

- help control cholesterol level
- prevent blood clotting, enhance platelet function
- prevent breast cancer and fibrocystic breast disease
- strengthen the lining of the arteries, i.e., protect against coronary artery disease
- strengthen the immune system
- protect against pollutants in the air
- protect against cataracts and retinal degeneration
- protect against arthritis and leg cramps

Good food sources of vitamin E are olive oil and wheat germ.

The research that's been done on cataract prevention with treatment of vitamin E makes a very strong case for this wonderful antioxidant. If we all lived long enough, we'd all get cataracts. This is because the lens of the eye, constantly subjected to the light of the sun and oxygen in the air, is extremely susceptible to a breakdown of the cell membrane as oxygen is transferred through the lipids that make up the structure of the outside of the cell. In human and animal studies, the correlation between antioxidant status and incidence of cataracts has been dramatically demonstrated. Although taking vitamin E won't prevent cataracts entirely (especially if you live a very long life), it will significantly delay their formation.

Drs. Robertson, Donner, and Trevithick[2] have done studies that indicate that the risk of forming cataracts was reduced by at least 50 percent in those individuals who took supplementary vitamins C and E.

And according to Dr. A. Taylor[3] and his colleagues at the U.S.D.A. Nutrition Research Center on Aging at Tufts University, delaying cataract formation by only ten years would eliminate the need for half the cataract extractions performed in the United States today.

Now that you understand the way free-radical damage works, it won't surprise you to learn that vitamin E can intervene in other disease patterns. Research on the effect of vitamin E on various medical conditions indicates that an abundance of E protects against free-radical damage that can destroy the body's tissues. For example, pigs on a regimen of vitamins E and C suffered much milder myocardial infarctions and recovered from them more quickly than rats that had not been supplemented with these vitamins. Rats pretreated with vitamin E had fewer symptoms of induced Parkinson's disease. There is clear laboratory evidence that vitamin E can be helpful in the treatment of chronic alcohol abuse.[4] It's been shown that rats that were fed alcohol, and as a result developed severe liver damage, have reduced levels of vitamin E because free-radical production occurs during the metabolism of alcohol in the body. The level of vitamin E has been shown to be lower in the blood of those pregnant women who develop preeclampsia, a potentially fatal condition of the last trimester. This offers a good reason to supplement pregnant women with vitamin E.[5]

Vitamin E even protects athletes from oxidative stress. As you may imagine, the harder you exercise, the greater the amount of oxygen you consume, the greater the loss of membrane function throughout the body. Dr. Meydani from Tufts University had two groups of exercising adults, one aged 22 to 35, the other aged 51 to 71, consume 400 IUs of vitamin E daily (my recommended dosage) for 48 days and found that even the older subjects, who are at greater risk of oxidative damage, were also protected by vitamin E.[6]

SELENIUM

Selenium is a trace element that occurs naturally in the soil and water in some regions. Some parts of the United States are selenium rich; some selenium poor. It's been found that people living in areas where natural selenium is plentiful (South Dakota has the highest rates) have a lower cancer mortality rate than those in areas where the soil lacks this trace element (Ohio has the lowest rates).

Selenium strengthens the immune system by producing more antibodies. It encourages phagocyte activity in the body—these are the protective cells that eat and absorb bacteria, viruses, and certain cancer cells.

It has been found that when selenium is mixed with vitamin E, their effects dovetail to give even greater protection to the body's immune system. Together, they produce a strong antioxidant reaction that can be invaluable as a retardant of the aging process. When taken together, selenium and vitamin E

- protect against tissue damage
- reduce symptoms of shingles
- reduce asthma attacks
- protect against stroke and heart disease
- reduce risk of cancers of the colon and pancreas

Since most food sources of selenium are very high in protein—tuna fish, codfish, chicken breast—I recommend that you consume selenium primarily from supplementation.

Dr. Anthony T. Diplock[7] has stated that selenium has been shown to prevent cancer in animals at high dosages. But it is considered safe for humans at lower dosages of 200 to 400 micrograms daily.

CALCIUM

Strong bones and teeth are formed throughout our life by a balanced exchange of the mineral calcium between our bones and our bloodstream. Our hormonal systems are greatly responsible for the laying down of calcium into bone tissue—they also prevent it from being reabsorbed into the bloodstream. But after 35, we start to lose bone mass. Women may actually lose as much as 30 to 50 percent of their total bone mass by the time they're 80. If they contract osteoporosis, a condition also known as "brittle" or "porous" bones, they may suffer from bone breaks that just won't heal. Osteoporosis currently affects 25 million people in the United States. Since most of us don't drink three to five eight-ounce glasses of milk or its equivalent daily, calcium supplements are essential, particularly for women over 50 or those of any age at high risk for osteoporosis.

Calcium carbonate supplements of 1,000 to 1,500 milligrams daily have been shown to slow bone loss in the hip and wrist.

Calcium also protects against colon cancer. In a study by Dr. Cedric Garland at the University of California at San Diego,[8] 25,620 individuals were tested for vitamin levels and incidence of colon cancer, and it was found that those with calcium serum levels of at least 20 milligrams per milliliter had 70 percent less risk of colon cancer.

Although new evidence[9] indicates that one particular gene's mutation may be responsible for colon cancer, calcium—along with vitamin E and selenium—can act as a powerful stabilizer to keep such cell changes from happening. Since vitamin D is necessary for calcium absorption, it's essential to consume 200 IU of D daily.

Even those with colon cancer may have a startling improvement with calcium supplementation. Dr. Freda Arlow, director of a study at the Veterans' Affairs Medical Center in Allen Park, Michigan, and Dr. Michael Wargovich, who did several studies at the University of Texas M. D. Anderson Cancer Center in Houston, Texas, recently found that, in patients who had a history of colorectal carcinoma, colon cancer cells were inhibited from proliferating after one to three months' daily supplementation of 1,500 to 2,000 milligrams of calcium.[10]

BETA CAROTENE

This antioxidant is a precursor or earlier form of vitamin A and is sometimes known as provitamin A. But unlike vitamin A, it presents no risks at high doses and, in fact, assists the body in producing its own form of vitamin A.

Beta carotene creates the brilliant fall foliage we so admire as well as the bright pink color of a flamingo's feathers and the extraordinary shades of tropical fish. As an edible quantity, it's present first and foremost in carrots, but it's also in other yellow fruits and vegetables—cantaloupes, papaya, oranges, yellow squash, and sweet potatoes.

Like selenium, beta carotene's function as an antioxidant for cancer prevention dovetails with that of vitamin E. Like vitamin E, it is fat soluble and therefore can do its work on fat-containing cell membranes. It has been shown to be enormously effective at trapping precancerous free radicals by gobbling up wild oxygen ions. It also provides a screen against the harmful ultraviolet rays of sunlight and other sources of radiation.

Recent research by Dr. Charles Hennekens, of Brigham and Women's Hospital in Boston, Massachusetts, who directed a six-year-study on 22,000 male physicians, indicates that beta carotene may also substantially reduce the risk of heart problems. Over a six-year period, the participants were randomly given either beta carotene in pill form, aspirin, a placebo, or a combination of those three every other day. Those 333 individuals with evidence of coronary artery disease who were given the beta carotene supplements had 50 percent fewer heart attacks, strokes, and other cardiac events than those taking a placebo.[11]

The good news is that beta carotene is readily available and you don't have to go to the health food store to get it. One carrot or one cantaloupe a day will give you the competitive edge on the aging process and may even protect you from heart disease. Other good food sources are peanuts, baked potatoes, and prunes.

I recommend the following daily dosages:

• Vitamin C: 1,000 milligrams in timed-release doses. Since vitamin C is excreted in the urine, you can lose a lot of its

benefit if you take it all at once. For extra effectiveness, you can divide this dose in thirds and take one portion with each meal.
- Vitamin E: 400 IU a day
- Selenium: 200 micrograms a day of yeast-free sodium selenite. Another selenium extract you may find for sale, known as seleno-methionine, has been implicated in elevated liver enzymes in extremely sensitive patients, so I advise you to stay away from it.
- Calcium:
  —Children under age 11, take 800 milligrams
  —For ages 11 to 24, take 1,200 milligrams
  —For ages 24–40 and for men over 40, take 800 milligrams
  —Pregnant or nursing women, 1,200 milligrams
  —Women over 40, take 1,200 to 1,500 milligrams. Use the higher value if you're in a high-risk category for osteoporosis, i.e., thin and small boned, fair haired, a heavy smoker, no longer producing estrogen because of a surgical menopause, or a family history of osteoporosis.
- Beta carotene: 6.6 milligrams a day, or one carrot, or one cantaloupe

In addition, the following may also be effective in treating certain diseases:

Supplement	My Recommended Daily Amount	Protects Against
lysine	400 mg.	herpes
pyridoxine (B-6)	25 mg.	PMS, carpal tunnel syndrome, immune deficiency
vitamin A	5,000 IU	heart disease, certain cancers
fiber	3.5 grams	colon cancer, high cholesterol
fish oil	3,000 mg.	heart disease, shingles
vitamin D with calcium	400 IU	osteoporosis
vitamin B-12	100 mcg.	anemia, neurological disease, depression

Making the Best Use of Your Life Expectancy

Every species on earth has its own typical life expectancy. We're all given a certain amount of energy to use, and the rate at which our bodies can repair damage to our DNA—the blueprint of life—gives us the maximum amount of time we're going to enjoy on earth.

But none of us ever really use our potential to the maximum. Most of us only utilize about one tenth of the brain power we're born with. Even Albert Einstein, it's said, consumed only a fifteenth of his. As those brain cells die off daily, we lose more and more of our capacity.

Of course, we don't have any conscious control over the chemical energy at our disposal. Some cells are able to regenerate; others are gone for good when they deteriorate. As we age, it's increasingly more difficult for our bodies to make new cellular life. And damage from cross linking and free-radicals reactions is impossible to avoid entirely.

But the energy you do have can last an amazingly long time if you treat your body right. By reducing the protein in your diet and by supplementing what you eat with the appropriate vitamins and trace minerals, you can undergo a process of rejuvenation and renewal, making yourself almost impervious to disease, strengthening your immune system, and synchronizing your internal and external states until they function as smoothly as the movement of a fine watch.

Part Three

How the Anti-Aging Diet Works

Chapter 9

Extending Your Own Life Span

Everyone is born, inhabits the earth for a limited amount of time, and then dies. For the past 100,000 years, man's life span has not stretched significantly—though in the past hundred years, since the advent of public health and antiseptic surgery and inoculation against major epidemics, more of us have been able to live out that one hundred-or-so years to which we are entitled.

Physical aging happens—I can't deny that. There are those who say that *mental aging* happens at a similar rate, and it sometimes happens more quickly, as in the case of Alzheimer's disease, where the mental process degenerates before the physical. However, there are measures we can take on both fronts, and they are relatively easy ones. The key is that we must start taking them now, in our thirties and forties. Let's look at the physical process first.

The Human Body in Flux

There are a variety of theories—and I don't completely buy any one of them—about why we start declining physically after 35 or so, and why after 65 it seems inevitable that we grow old. One is that each of our cells is programmed for a certain set period of years, and winds down like a clock. Another is that we undergo so much damage from free radicals and oxidation that our bodies eventually break down. And a third is the molecular confusion theory—that mistakes start happening in the interactions between different cells, that they mutate and change faster as they grow older until, finally, they don't even recognize each other. And because all systems in the body depend on other systems, if they can't communicate, they can't self-perpetuate.

Regardless of which theory or combination of theories you subscribe to, the end result is that the aging process begins the moment you arrive in the world. Many of your cells—those in the skin, for example—are lost at such an enormous rate that they have to be replaced, but the rest of you is slowly but surely degenerating from day one. You lose about fifty thousand nerve cells a day, and they can never regrow—your body cannot manufacture new ones. An infant female has about two million eggs in her ovaries, but by the time she's a grown woman, she has only about eight thousand left and only three hundred or four hundred menstrual cycles in which to give any of those a fighting chance at conception.

As the body ages, it doesn't function as efficiently as it used to, and the various organs don't have as much capacity or reserve. After 35, the various systems just don't perform at their peak. By the age of 85, you can expect:

- your reaction time to slow 15 percent
- your heart output to decline 40 percent
- your bone mass to decline 30 to 50 percent
- your kidney function to decline 30 percent
- your kidney blood flow to decline 55 percent
- your maximum breathing capacity to decline 65 percent

If you reach the age of 100, you will more than likely experience:

- arterial wall rigidity
- cataract formation
- graying and thinning of your hair

- loss of kidney reserve
- loss of elasticity of your skin

Yes? True? Well, it's true if you don't make any effort to change that. If you pay no attention to diet, exercise, or the way you feel about getting older, you certainly will age.

But the good news is this: it doesn't have to be this way. You can change your destiny! And you can change it dramatically.

You do have a choice in your own aging process, and I'm going to tell you just how to make it.

How the Anti-Aging Diet Can Retard the Aging Process

The wonderful news about eating a low-protein diet is that, in fact, you can disprove all the scientific theory. You can show up all those medical practitioners and laboratory scientists who say there's nothing that can be done about aging.

The crucial factor here is plasticity. If something is "plastic," it's moveable, changeable, variable. And, thank heavens, that's what human life and potential is.

You can't play around with extending the human life span and, for this reason, scientists who are examining life extension alter the various habits of rats in a laboratory. Drs. Ross, Lustbader, and Bras of the Fox Chase Cancer Center, in Philadelphia, Pennsylvania, and the University of Utrecht, the Netherlands, posited that dietary habits could make a significant difference in predicting the life span of rats. "Nutrition, by modulating the changes that occur in a living system with passage of time, is recognized to be a significant environmental factor that can influence longevity."[1]

Since McCay's early experiments in the 1930s,[2] food restriction has been the method of extending rats' lives—often doubling their normal life expectancy with the additional benefit of eliminating age-related diseases. But an interesting study by Dr. Byung Pal Yu at the University of Texas Health Science Center, San Antonio, showed that restricting protein without restricting calories produced a 10 to 15 percent increase in longevity, and that by also reducing calorie intake could lengthen life span by as much as 50 percent![3]

Rats lead a simple life guided by the sure hand of laboratory researchers. We, on the other hand, live extraordinarily complex lives. We can't just let nature take its course—we've got to work to alter our destiny. And it's not difficult.

You can make a personal effort to change your life-style now and feel great when you're 100. It's up to you.

Making Choices

If you decide, at the age of 35, that you want to live to 120, you will have to make a personal effort to do this. You are going to have to take steps to alter what nature wants to do, which is to age you at the statistically correct rate for your chronological years.

The following listing shows the amazing number of factors that are within your control:

THE TEN COMMANDMENTS

1. Reduce the protein in your diet now—and for the rest of your life.

2. Exercise moderately today, and tomorrow and every day for the rest of your life.

3. Stop smoking. Enough has been written on this subject; suffice it to say that destroying your lungs and reducing the amount of oxygen available to your brain are suicidal pursuits. If you've just quit, congratulations—and don't start up again if you value your life.

4. Stop indulging in recreational drugs—or don't start.

5. Reduce alcohol consumption to one drink a week, if that.

Biomarkers of Aging

One of the chief goals of the Anti-Aging Diet is to stretch you physiologically so that your biological age can be twenty to thirty years younger than your chronological age.

Most of us have much more control over our body's aging rate than we think. It's always amazing to me to meet people I would place somewhere between 60 years and death and find that they're my age—but I'm never surprised to hear that they also drink, smoke, and lead a sedentary life. Although genetics certainly does affect the aging process, there's a great deal more that goes into it. And every one of us can make changes in our biological time clock *if we want to.*

Researchers have come up with some interesting standard tests to determine the rate of the aging process.[4] These particular factors seem to change subtly over the years—and yet, in the presence of good health and the absence of disease, the biomarkers can remain very similar, even though the chronological age of the person tested increases.

OF ANTI-AGING

6. Stay out of the sun. Sunlight is responsible for 90 percent of the aging of your skin.

7. See a doctor once a year for a checkup. If you see your physician when you're healthy, you may never have to see him when you're ill. This is a vital part of life extension by preventive medicine.

8. Ask your doctor to teach you how to practice breast, testicular, and skin self-exams and practice them on a regular basis.

9. Learn about methods of safer sex and always practice them.

10. Get six to eight hours sleep a night to give your body and mind rest and recovery time.

The tests measure:

- fingertip sensitivity
- memory
- pulmonary function
- hearing
- visual acuity
- movement time

Fingertip sensitivity is related to the responses of the circulatory and nervous systems. The more sensitive an individual in feeling something placed on the tip of his finger, the younger his circulatory and nervous systems are judged to be.

Memory loss has long been associated with the aging process. If your different memory functions barely change even as you get older—when brain cells are no longer being replaced and neurotransmitter connections are being made less rapidly—you are biologically younger than your years.

Pulmonary function, or the capacity of your lungs to expand and hold oxygen, is lost as you age at approximately 10 percent per decade after the age of 30. By the age of 70, you may have lost about 40 percent of your original lung capacity. If, however, you exercise regularly and keep your lung tissue active and elastic, your pulmonary function will decline much less rapidly.

Hearing begins to decline at age 40; hearing loss levels off about age 65. Abuse of your hearing function can be caused by attending loud rock concerts, living in the midst of a noisy city, being subject to loud noises like gunshots, and so on. But by avoiding some of the major hearing offenses, you can greatly reduce the level of average decline.

Visual acuity begins to decline at age 40; it levels off about age 65. Genetics play a big part in the biological age of your eyes, but certain vitamins can truly prevent some of the natural disease processes that affect your vision as you age (see Chapter 8).

Movement time represents how mobile a person is, how well and how quickly he can get up from a chair, climb a flight of stairs, or walk a mile. The faster you're able to move, the younger you are.

Are You Younger or Older Than Your Age?

If you're currently a 45-year-old woman, your life expectancy was 77.9 at your birth. But today, having survived this long, you can expect to live to 82.8. Women tend to live six years longer than men, until you get up into your mid-eighties and the expectancies become almost equal. As people get healthier, the odds get even better. According to the U.S. Department of the Census, at its most recent count in 1989, there were nearly 54,000 individuals over 100 in the country—that's a huge leap from only 12,000 in 1979. And by the year 2,000, it's projected that there will be over five million individuals over the age of 85 in the United States.

Some of us have a particular genetic propensity for survival. If your grandparents were going strong at 80 or 90, there's a very good chance that your parents will—and that you will, too. If, on the other hand, you come from a family where several relatives died of heart disease or cancer or some other life-threatening ailment, you may be predisposed to that condition. Even then, you can lower your risk significantly by changing your life-style.

But how old you are and how old you feel can be two entirely different things. We all know some young person who's been through a devastating physical or emotional event who literally "ages" overnight. Their posture is stooped, their skin sallow, they have less energy than a person twice their age. I'd rather talk about the other end of the spectrum, though, where elderly people just refuse to act their age. They have spring in their step, an eagerness to explore new avenues—they even dress and talk differently from their peers.

I think a lot of factors come into play here. Being deeply committed to a job or avocation, having a close-knit circle of friends and relations, intimacy with another human being—sexual and affectionate—and having a generally positive outlook on life can take years off you.

Mind-Fitness Immunization

Now we'll examine the mental side of aging. Here we really have to combine mental and emotional acuity, because the attitude you have about life in general directly influences the thoughts you think about it.

There are those who look at a glass and say it's half empty. I always look at it as half full—maybe even a little more than half. This is my personal way of expressing my positive mental attitude toward life. And it's essential if you want a long and healthy existence.

Your perspective on life is often formed by past experiences, your current state of emotional well-being, and particularly by your expectations for the future. If those three elements can be strengthened and toned, just like your body, there is no reason in the world why you can't use that positive attitude to immunize yourself against hardship, trauma, boredom, and any misfortunes that may come your way.

TO BE MENTALLY AND EMOTIONALLY FIT, TRY FOLLOWING THESE SUGGESTIONS:

1. Never dwell on one particular problem for long periods of time or it will become too much of a focal point for negative feelings. Make lists of things that make you feel negative and try to examine them again, this time from a new angle.

2. Find some humor in every situation, no matter how bleak it seems.

3. Remember that "tincture of time" is the ultimate cure for many problems—it's fruitless to keep mulling a problem over and over, looking desperately for an answer, when only time will cure it.

If you can keep these three suggestions in mind, whatever is happening in your life will be more manageable.

I'm not suggesting that you overlook the unfortunate, the tragic, or the inevitable. I don't want you to turn into a Pollyanna who sees everything through rose-colored lenses. No, all I want to do is show you how to give yourself permission to enjoy every minute of the exceptionally long and healthy life you're going to have. For some, this may take some work. It's not always easy to look on the bright side. But it can and should be done, because getting your mind and spirit in shape may be the most important factor in successful living and aging.

The ancient science of alchemy was based on the belief that it's possible to combine simple things to create something really remarkable. Now it's time for you to turn straw into gold, dark into light, and negatives into positives with the element we call mind-fitness.

Your Mental Ability Can Grow as You Age

Some memory loss inevitably accompanies the aging process. In order to remember anything, the neurons in your brain must make certain connections with one another. If you forget something, the reason is probably that those connections have been severed. About 50,000 of our nerve cells die each day and don't replenish themselves; others shrink or lose their ability to make connections with other neurons. There are also chemical changes in brain tissue over time. Messengers known as neurotransmitters that are supposed to travel between one neuron and another to make connections begin to fluctuate in strength and capacity over time.

Finally, medications may interfere with memory. There are dozens of prescription and over-the-counter drugs that may severely hamper your brain's ability to retain information. When you've been on the anti-aging lifetime program for a few months, you may be able to reduce or eliminate most of your medications, with your doctor's approval. When you do, you'll not only function better physically but mentally as well.

A decline in mental alertness associated with aging has been linked to a slower central nervous system, the result of less oxygen traveling to the brain. But regular exercise can increase the circulation and result in a quicker reaction time as well as better memory.

There are three different types of memory. Long-term memory—a car accident in your childhood or your wedding day—is engraved on your mind forever. Primary memory, which involves the ability to repeat a phone number or the items on a shopping list right after hearing or seeing them, is designed for immediate use and remains about the same no matter how old we are. Secondary or short-term memory, which includes information such as where you parked your car at the mall or recalling the items on your list an hour after you read it, is increasingly more difficult to retain as you age.

If you've started noticing some mental slips, don't get down about it. Just because you can't remember the names of your daughter's five new friends doesn't mean you're losing your mind. By all means, keep a positive attitude about your mental ability. If you forget something and spend a lot of time beating yourself up about it, it can be a self-perpetuating pattern. Be confident that tomorrow, what seemed hard to remember will slide effortlessly into place for you.

No matter how old you are, there are mental exercises you can do to improve your memory. Your ability to learn new things can grow as you get older, and just as you can strengthen your body with exercise, so you can also work your brain into a better, fitter shape.

Use these mental toning exercises often:

1. Practice using mnemonic devices. Medical students traditionally get through memorizing long lists of bones by making up a sentence whose words use the same initial letters as the names on the list. "Wriggling snakes are not too popular" could help you recall that you need watermelon, salad greens, apples, a notepad, tissues, and pasta at the market.

2. Practice associating names with concrete images. If you're introduced to Mary Cohen, try to conjure up an image of Mary leading her little lamb wearing a big pointed cone on her head.

3. Look for landmarks. When you park your car, look at the store next to it, the shape of the tree beside it, and so on. If you have nothing to go by but the number in the lot, say, B-30, you might think about what you were doing on your thirtieth birthday.

4. Use rhymes to make associations. If you can't recall that you need cheese and plums, you might think of "please come."

5. Try to make associations between the disconnected items you have to remember and places they might logically go. For the cheese, think of a mousehole; you could imagine milk near the front door where the milkman once might have left it.

If you work on these techniques daily, taking a conscious and active role in toning your brain cells, you may never notice a decline in your mental fitness, regardless of your age.

How to Change Your Attitude Toward Aging

A journey begins with just one step, the Chinese say. When you're preparing for a long life, you have all the time in the world to get to your ultimate goal.

As with your diet and exercise changes, you will find that the less you do, the more you accomplish simply by making small, positive changes in the way you approach a problem. You don't need to change your job, move to Fiji, or meditate two hours a day. All you have to do is become aware of yourself and of some of your typical reactions to stress or hardship.

- Identify your problems
- Prioritize—decide what to do first
- Manage your time better—leave time for things you really want to do, or feel you should do well
- Try new tactics on old problems
- Spend time with supportive rather than negative people

You will be delighted to see after only a few weeks that this body/mind connection is working, slowly but subtly. If you understand that each cell is a sentient entity, with its own potential for "wanting" to go on, "wanting" to live longer, you'll understand a little about how these two systems are growing together.

Mind and Body Together

A variety of interesting tests has indicated that the more fit your mind is, the more immunized against disease your body can be. Wanting to be healthy can actually keep you from contracting any one of the over two hundred viruses we are exposed to on a regular basis. Your immune system is positively reinforced by diet and exercise and mental attitude.

Go back and take the quiz entitled "How Fit Is Your Mind?" in

Chapter 1. You may notice, now that you've been on the Anti-Aging Diet and exercise plan for a while, that, though you haven't consciously thought about it, you have "changed your mind." As your body has begun to get into shape and grow younger, you feel better about yourself. You've proven to yourself how much you're capable of and can see that you can go beyond where you are now. Having lost weight, your clothes fit; you can cross your legs again. Having made your mind more fit, you're better able to deal with stresses as challenges instead of obstacles. They are now your most creative opportunities.

As you can do more, you can be more. And it will only come naturally in this course of events that you will want the maximum amount of time in which to accomplish all your goals. You don't need to retire, you don't need to stop dreaming, you don't need to age.

Look beyond today to the future. It's your birthday, and you're 100 years old, you feel wonderful, and you have myriad possibilities ahead of you.

Chapter 10

The Essential Truth of Anti-Aging

You need only one more ingredient in my breakthrough anti-aging program, one which will allow you to create your own "fountain of youth" and make it your own.

The truth that has driven thinkers and explorers from Ponce de Leon to New Age life-extension gurus is right in front of you. Like most extraordinary finds, it's as complex as it is simple; as simple as it is complex.

You cannot slow the aging process and improve the quality of the extra years you're going to have with a pill, a magic formula, a new vaccine, a rejuvenation cream, or a trip to a mystical hot spring beneath some ancient Indian ruins. But you can make a difference by relying on the combination of elements you've just added to your life—the diet, exercise, vitamins and minerals, and positive mental attitude.

The truth involves the way you live your life and what you expect of yourself as the years pass. So learn it and emblazon it on your heart:

If you never quit, if you always create a new challenge, a new goal for yourself, you will remain young forever. No matter what your age, if you have the will and energy to keep motivated, busy, and involved, your life will become an endless banquet of excitement and variety. Best of all, you'll never be bored, even if you live to be 120.

Where Does 40 Fit in the Scheme of Things?

It's upsetting to me to hear a young patient tell me he feels old. Yet there are so many people out there who are bored at 30, exhausted at 40, and can't begin to imagine the benefits of living to 100. If you find yourself in this category, let me tell you something—the ground-breaking effects of the Anti-Aging Diet are going to alter your attitude about where you fit in the scheme of things, just as they have for thousands of my patients at the Southwest Health Institute.

Remember that the baby boomers are all cumulatively going to live longer than the last generation did. This means that seniors of the twenty-first century are going to play a much larger part in society. They are going to take their rightful place in the Western world that they have so long enjoyed in the Far East. They will be the voices of reason and experience and, as such, will be able to help shape the ideas of younger people.

Then, too, you can think about the benefits you'll be reaping of not just years but decades of preventive health measures you're taking now. By sticking with the Anti-Aging Diet, your regular exercise program, a sensible regimen of vitamins and minerals, and the additional positive effects of thinking and feeling youthful, your quality of life will improve with the years.

Aging is *not* a disease. It is a process, ongoing from the day you were born.

Think of the way your body and mind started changing in your early teens. You were confused, excited, half child and half adult. The same may be true when you're in your thirties and forties. You are midway through your life, and you have the capacity to go in many directions. This is the time, with your experience and maturity, to make sure you're setting yourself up for "someday."

By sticking with your anti-aging lifetime program, you can:

• agree not to settle for anything and embark on new adventures every day
• reduce the risk of the physical and emotional effects of mid-life crisis, because the life you're leading won't give you any opportunity for regrets about what you should have done
• alleviate the threat and anxiety of lonely years after divorce or the death of a spouse because you'll have the attitude necessary to start over each time you reach a setback
• minimize the risk of depression now by enjoying your new-found abilities and energies so that you won't be faced with the fear of being a depressed older person

Plan Your Future Now

Think about all the things you never have time to do now. Start making a list and add to it on a weekly basis. You may think of small goals, like growing a fig tree in your backyard or building a boat in a bottle. Or you may have large ones, like starting up a new career or becoming so involved in an activity that is currently an avocation that it becomes a second job. If you give it some real thought, you may surprise yourself at what you come up with.

I am constantly impressed and overwhelmed by my patients' thoughts about the future. I originally asked them to think up a few practical but challenging five-year plans—things they'd always felt they might like to do if they had the time. But most of them came back to me with much, more more. Here are samples of some of the ten-year, twenty-year, and someday plans my patients have come up with. Maybe these will spark some ideas of your own.

Ten-Year Plans

go back to school
write or paint

volunteer at a hospital

start a barbershop quartet (or a rock group) and get bookings

run a marathon

get elected to the local school board

become involved in city-run urban renovation for low-income
    housing

join a community theater group

start a limited day-care facility at home

Twenty-Year Plans

travel

tutor illiterate adults or troubled children

start selling the crafts you make (jewelry, quilting) at local fairs
    and on consignment in stores

teach a class in something you know well at your local YMCA

hire yourself out as a speaker on any topic you know a lot
    about

Someday Plans

build homes for the homeless

work for the Red Cross in underdeveloped countries

bike around the United States

learn how to do organic farming

invent something and patent it

get involved in an environmental project to help save the
    earth

A New Focus: Outward Instead of Inward

An interesting fact surfaces in every interview of extraordinary
individuals who live actively into extreme advanced age: they all

devote a good deal of their intensity and energy to something bigger than they are. Their delight in each new day has a lot to do with an unselfish ability to look beyond the petty and personal.

There is no reason to wait until you're 80 to develop this facility. Now is the time to make good friends and learn to do for them, not just for you. I'm not suggesting that you should become a saint. What I'm talking about here is a way of projecting yourself into the world. Your early and middle years of career development, of making and raising a family, tend to focus you on personal concerns—and so they should. But you can be more, and you'll find that you're a happier person if you commit yourself to some goal beyond today—beyond just you.

This commitment doesn't have to be anything earth shattering. Your goal can be a mural you've always wanted to paint, a trip around the world, a volunteer job at a hospital. When I interview patients who appear younger than their chronological age, they're always involved in something (or a few somethings) whether they're 80 or 95 years old. The French call it a *raison d'être*, which translates as "a reason for being." When you've got that challenge in front of you, the extra years become a bonus instead of an onus.

Think about changing your ideas about leisure time now—leisure is time to actively do what you want, not time to do nothing.

Being a Social Animal

People need people. Social stimulation gives you an edge, someone to bounce your ideas off, someone to eat with, talk with, walk with. If you have no one, you have less of a reason to stay well, to look good, to live a long time. Not that your own company can't be enjoyable, but the lack of company can be a terrible burden. And one of the greatest fears about growing older is loneliness.

Everyone needs the support of friends and family, but particularly as we age. Our parents and their friends can be assets to us—and to our own children. And as we baby boomers get older, we'll be able to see this from the other side—we can nurture the next generation, and they can serve as a rejuvenating force for us.

Changing Your Concept of Aging

It's up to you to change society's idea of what "old" means, or rather, to return to the original meaning of the word. In Old English, *eald* means "to grow, nourish, to bring up," and the Greek cognate *analfos* means "insatiable." What a concept for the next generation, that the elderly will be insatiable in their thirst for good health, new and varied experience, and the right to be leaders of their society.

In an informal survey conducted while writing this book, I asked people in different age groups and from different economic backgrounds how long they wanted to live and how their feelings about aging reflected their own or society's attitudes. Most respondents were deeply influenced by other older people they had known. Those who had lived with a vital grandparent or who had been friendly with an older person who loved life were very much looking forward to their own period of less stress and more time to do just what they wanted. These people, who ranged in age from 19 to 55, hoped to live between 80 and 100 years, in a country setting, with a spouse or sibling.

On the other hand, those respondents who had experienced a very negative attitude toward aging from their own parents, or who had a grandparent in a nursing care facility, were doubtful about living much past 70. One such respondent answered, "I'd like to live to 60, or as long as I have my health and all my marbles."

I'm telling you now: Don't think about Aunt Millie in the nursing home. Assume that this woman never took care of her mind and body, that she was overly dependent on medication, and that she lost the will to live well after she was forced to retire from her job at 65. She has nothing to do with the way you will age!

I think one of the best growing experiences we can have is to learn the range and depth of our mental and physical abilities as well as our limitations. I've learned so much from patients of mine who've been through major illnesses or injuries and seem to have a spark that cannot be extinguished. I've known former athletes who can't compete anymore because of physical restrictions but who are not discouraged by their new limitations. They simply change their goals. Instead of aiming for a marathon, they can work toward good levels of daily exercise that will keep their cardiovascular, respiratory, and musculoskeletal systems in excellent shape.

As for the positive attitude, that's something that must also be nourished and developed over the years—another muscle to get in shape.

When you've revised your concept of aging so that it's realistically shaped by the way you take care of yourself today and intend to in the future, you should go back to the longevity quiz in the first chapter of this book (page 14) and take it again. See how far you've come! Why shouldn't you want to work till you're 80 and then enjoy yourself for another twenty or thirty years? You'll have experience, wisdom, and maturity behind you. You'll also have been able to save more money by earning an income for fifteen or twenty additional years so that when you do stop working—we're not going to call it retirement—you can have an easier life-style with more benefits and more respect.

Believe me, the image of what elderly implies is going to change if more of us live to 100 and do it well. Just by sticking around and being there as role models, we'll spread a more enlightened view of the benefits inherent in aging.

Older people have something you can't buy for any amount of money, and that's experience. They've seen changes over time; they've helped to make those changes. This gives people with a lot of years under their belt a vast perspective on our country, our future, our children, our economic and political life, and our environment. Preserving the planet means preserving people, too.

A Few Case Histories

Let me tell you about some of my patients who are shining examples of the way we can all relish the extraordinary benefits of our prospective longevity.

I start with my own wife Molly, because she's got the attitude I'm talking about. At 32, Molly is a breathtakingly beautiful woman (much more so than she was at 20, by the way), a wife, mother, stepmother, and actress and singer. In a profession where generally only the very young survive and those past 30 (except, of course, for Mick Jagger and Bonnie Raitt!) are looked on by record executives as on the downslide, Molly is on the upswing. She tells me that the low-protein life-style, which she's been following for the past four years, has made a radical difference in the way she looks at herself and her career. When she's on tour in Europe or America, she's not jet lagged; she's ready to go. In a recording studio, the pressures and hassles don't get to her. She knows that aging is another credit on her resume, along with the increasingly long list of television shows, movies, and concert dates.

She has been told that her voice is taking on more mature and interesting colors; she's getting all sorts of different parts now, thanks to her talent and hard work, and especially thanks to her increased experience and devotion to her career. She loves life and, therefore, people treat her as though she deserves the best kind of life. It's a cyclical process, she says, and a totally rewarding one.

Now, let me tell you about a patient of mine who's a little older than Molly but has that same zest for life. Reuben is 91 years old, although he looks about 72. "If you take care of yourself and don't abuse yourself," Reuben states, "you can last a long time."

He has four orange trees in his yard, and he gets a lot of exercise picking the fruit he eats daily. He's switched to low-fat milk, eats much less protein than he used to, and has cut back on sweets in recent years, eating smaller portions of cake and pie. He gave up pipe smoking a long time ago and consumes alcohol only once or twice a year, on social occasions.

Reuben and his wife met at a dance sixty-six years ago, and they've been dancing ever since. They've cut back from four to two nights a week recently, once for square dancing and once for ballroom dancing. Reuben thinks he's moving around at least half of the four to five hours they're at the dance hall, and he's thinking all the time. "When they call those squares, you've got to know the steps. You can't sit down because others in your square depend on you."

Of his occasional aches and twinges, Reuben says, "When you hit 90, there's got to be something wrong with you, otherwise you're not normal." I can't for the life of me find anything wrong with this man—but everything right.

I've learned a lot from an attorney named Albert who came to see me at 34 so depressed he could hardly go to work in the morning. His success in the eyes of the world made no difference to him—he felt powerless to control his emotional volatility. Albert told me, when we first met, that he felt he was at the end. He'd done it all, seen it all, and he was sick and tired. A two-pack-a-day smoker and a heavy drinker, Albert had been diagnosed as a manic depressive and was taking Lithium to counteract his severe mood swings.

When I tell you it was a good thing that Albert had an addictive personality, I know you won't believe me. But his recovery was based on the fact that he and I were able to use his terrible condition for the good. He was easy to convince when I said he absolutely *had* to start a low-protein diet and daily exercise program. He became fanatic about both, rapidly lost twenty pounds, and saw an incredible drop in both cholesterol and blood pressure readings. The diet suppressed his desire for smoking, and he enjoyed running so much that he was motivated to work his way up to three miles a day.

But the greatest improvement in Albert can't be charted along with his clinical changes. Here was a man who thought it was all over at 34. Within just three months, he told me he knew he could live forever like this. He was looking forward to 50, to 60, and beyond. But, more important, he was looking forward to tomorrow.

Another favorite patient of mine is Florence, 87, a small, elegant woman, a retired psychologist, who dresses beautifully and carries herself like a queen. She'd had heart problems for years but certainly never expected to suffer a burst aneurysm in her aorta at the age of 82. She was alone in her apartment and fell to the floor, feeling as though she were "coming apart."

When she recovered, she decided that it was important to keep her focus off herself and on others. Now, the younger members of her building co-op come to her for advice. They depend on her, she tells me, so she has to stay in good shape and not let things get to her.

One of her best recommendations for health is meditation—she's been doing it to reduce stress for over twenty years. "I appear to be cool and collected," she says, "but I'm sometimes a mess inside, and this helps me calm down."

Don't you think, if we all woke up every day feeling as committed and excited about life as these individuals, that it would be a treat to live as long as we possibly could?

Living to Be Healthy and Wise . . . and Maybe Wealthy, Too

If you're active and the quality of your life is good, if you've been able to maintain a fit body and have practiced preventive care so that you never contract one of the diseases associated with aging, why not enjoy life as long as you possibly can? All you need is the right attitude about how long you will live, work, and play.

By the year 2040, Medicare costs for the oldest in our society— those over 85—will have increased sixfold from the current figure.[1] Projections for long-term health care are astronomical—way beyond the financial capacity of most Americans. It's going to be so expensive to get sick by the time you reach the next century, you'll simply have to stay well. On the other hand, with all the money you'll be saving on medical bills, you can probably go around the world or build a vacation home.

When you understand that what you do for yourself today can drastically affect the way you feel tomorrow, the future looks bright, indeed. When you have a body that's been on a low-protein diet for decades, you will circumvent conditions such as liver failure, kidney failure, gout, and arthritis as well as many types of cancer. When you have a body that's been walking or doing some other form of exercise for decades, you radically decrease the risk of cardiovascular and pulmonary diseases and osteoporosis.

If this healthy body does come down with something, it will heal quickly because its immune system will be so much stronger from the lifelong combination you've given it of diet, exercise, and mental fitness.

What Does Healthy Aging Entail?

This is not to say that you will be able to avoid all the changes that come with aging. Remember that aging, in and of itself, is not a disease. Healthy aging is a process of development that starts the day you're born. Maybe your legs will bother you in cold weather; maybe your hair will start thinning or you'll have a few varicose veins. But if you take care of yourself from your thirties and forties onward, you'll never have to cope with any life-threatening ailments.

Joseph Beasley and Jerry Swift, authors of *The Kellogg Report: The Impact of Nutrition, Environment and Lifestyle on the Health of Americans,* quote from Hoke, 1968:270 in the *Archives of Environmental Health:* "Health is not a static, platonic, ideal state nor only a homeostatic balance. Health is a form of behavior . . . 'doings' that are willed, or motivated, either consciously or unconsciously. They proceed *from* a person. Health, as behavior . . . is more like a character trait such as honesty. Honesty is not a goal in itself but is a method of pursuing other goals. In the same sense, health is not a static end point but a *way* of pursuing one's goals."[2]

Remember what Thomas Jefferson once said: "You should spend at least two hours a day on bodily exercise; however, if you should decide not to, you will someday spend two hours a day taking care of your disease."

Stay with the Anti-Aging Diet! This breakthrough program will not just make you slimmer and fitter, as it has done for thousands of my patients, but it will also increase the quality of the rest of your life, so that you can live each day with a new determination, a new goal ahead.

When you love life, you'll look younger, you'll smile and laugh more frequently, the furrows will gradually disappear from between your brows, your eyes will shine, and your energy level will skyrocket.

Other people will look at you in amazement and wonder what's going on. They'll want to emulate that good feeling you're spreading around and make it their own.

So now that you know the truth, don't keep it to yourself. Let it out, make it public knowledge! Share the principles of the Anti-Aging Diet with everyone. The more often you pass the truth on to others, the more indelibly etched it will become in your own mind, body, and soul.

Chapter 11

The Most Commonly Asked Questions About Aging and the Anti-Aging Diet

We are all curious about what it's going to be like when we get older. There are so many unknowns! How will we feel? What can we do and what can't we do? Will we even want to live longer than the statistical life expectancy?

Until you've reached and passed a life goal, you never really know what it's going to be like. We're all different, and aging affects us all differently. Some individuals feel and look just the same for decades. Others seem to have aged overnight. Why is this? And more important, how can you be one of those who feels as young at 90 as you do at 30?

Here are some of the most commonly asked questions about aging. As with every experience we haven't yet had, it's nice to have a head start on what it's going to be like when we get there.

Q: How long can our bodies really last?
A: We can live to 120 if we lead the right life-style and try not to abuse our bodies too badly. Anatomically, the body is designed to last this long, and historically there are civilizations whose members have lived even longer. Certainly our modern medical tech-

nology makes it possible for us not only to survive but to live well into later years. Only a negative or hopeless attitude about the future degrades the quality of life as we age.

Q: Is it true that, as I get older, I'm necessarily going to become more lonely?

A: It's really up to you. As more people live longer, there's going to be less loneliness because we're going to have our peers living right alongside us. A big key to warding off loneliness is participation in groups and especially getting involved with younger people. This not only helps to prevent loneliness but also slows the aging process because it stimulates and boosts your energy level. There are many options—you could join a church group or volunteer organization, maybe even start a new career after retirement. Or better yet . . . don't even think about retiring!

Q: Do facial creams really improve the appearance of your skin? And which ones are best?

A: Facial creams rehydrate the skin, improving appearance, though they cannot remove wrinkles. Creams containing the antioxidants vitamin E, selenium, and beta carotene will be the revolutionary breakthrough in twenty-first-century skin care.

Q: Can facials reduce aging?

A: Facials can't reverse the aging process. However, you tend to feel better about yourself after you've had one. You get more benefit from the impetus a facial gives you to take better care of your skin on an everyday basis than you derive from the actual chemicals that are applied to your face.

Q: Can chemical peels and dermabrasion restore my skin to a more youthful condition?

A: Chemical peels can remove fine lines but not deep wrinkles. Depending on the chemical used and the depth of the burn your skin receives, you will have to repeat the process when the skin grows back, a matter of months in most cases. Peeling should only be done by estheticians, plastic surgeons, or dermatologists because phenol—the abrasive peeling acid—can be dangerous if the practitioner is not skilled in its use.

Q: Is there a loss of libido as we get older?
A: Men and women in their nineties can have a satisfactory sex life; certainly people in their eighties can enjoy sex several times a week if they wish. The intensity of their libido depends on their diet and exercise program and often on any medications they may be taking. For example, beta blockers and hypertensives, antidepressants, and tranquilizers may depress the libido and lower desire. Vaginal creams with estrogen or estrogen taken orally can increase vaginal lubrication. These must be prescribed by your physician. There are other, over-the-counter lubricants—K-Y jelly replens, and Astroglide—that mimic the natural secretions of the body.

Q: Will I still be able to enjoy sex after menopause?
A: Absolutely. You may require additional lubricants and you and your partner may both require more time for arousal and climax, but there is no reason you can't have the same frequency of and delight in sex you always had.

Q: My grandfather lived to 95. Will I?
A: There certainly are genetic markers, and the likelihood of living to advanced old age is stronger if you come from a family where everyone lived a long time. However, you can alter your own life expectancy greatly by the way you live. If you smoke, eat a high-protein diet, and abuse alcohol or drugs, you can easily cancel out the predisposition of your good genes. On the other hand, even if no one in your family had the genes for long life, you can extend your own existence with a proper diet, a regular exercise program, and a positive mental attitude.

Q: If I live a very long life, will I eventually be blind and deaf?
A: In the natural course of aging, you lose about 10 percent of your sense of smell, taste, sight, and hearing, but the loss levels off. If you're 40 and have high-frequency hearing loss, that doesn't

mean you'll be deaf by the time you're 60. You may need glasses at 40, but you won't necessarily need bifocals in ten more years.

The chances of cataract development increase with age—if you live to 100, you may well develop one. However, taking the anti-oxidants vitamins C and E from midlife on may well protect the lenses of your eyes.

Q: Will I lose my taste for food as I age?
A: Older people often complain that their food is tasteless, and they consequently add more salt and sugar to their diet. But this is frequently due to overmedication and lack of exercise. Tastebuds do not necessarily change or decline during the aging process.

Q: What are liver spots?
A: Senile purpura, known as liver spots, are discolorations due to thinning of the skin—you grow fewer new layers of epidermis as you age. Sometimes these spots may be related to capillary fragility. Your capillaries become more fragile over time, and as they break down you experience increased bleeding into the skin. Unfortunately, no miracle creams will erase or prevent these spots. However, since photoaging is the major contributory factor, stay out of the sun! Incidentally, these marks have no link to your liver function, despite their name.

Q: Do I have to stop sunbathing because I'm getting older?
A: You should never have started! Prolonged exposure to the ultraviolet rays of the sun should be avoided. There is a drastic increase in the rate of malignant melanoma or skin cancer in America, linked to the amount of sun exposure received prior to age 18.

Q: I've heard great things about minoxidol for hair growth. Should I use it on my thinning hair?
A: Minoxidol has proved effective for some people, but it takes three to four months to see any result, and you must use the product continuously for the rest of your life to rejuvenate your hair follicles and maintain new growth. It is also a very expensive treatment. If you're determined to improve your hair, you might make

a better investment in hair transplants and other restoration methods. Not every man loses his hair as he ages, but there is a genetic predisposition to male pattern baldness. Remember, there is nothing wrong with being bald—many women find baldness attractive and sexy; only men seem to regard it as a terrible sign of aging.

Women who experience hair loss after menopause find it particularly distressing. The hair loss is sometimes caused by hormonal changes; however, it can be caused by an underactive thyroid gland. For this reason, hair loss should be evaluated by your doctor.

Q: Am I in danger of contracting osteoporosis as I get older?
A: This condition, known as "porous" or "brittle" bones, most commonly develops in postmenopausal women who are at higher risk if they are blond, fair-skinned, thin smokers who never exercise. This is a "silent" disease—you don't know you have osteoporosis until you break a bone and it proves difficult or impossible to heal. But if you take care of yourself in your twenties and thirties, when your bone growth is at its peak, you will lower your chances of developing osteoporosis, despite being in a high-risk category. Stop smoking, engage in weight-bearing exercise, and eat a diet high in calcium. If you are postmenopausal, you may wish to consider estrogen supplementation (hormone replacement therapy) after consultation with your doctor. Estrogen prevents calcium from being reabsorbed into the bloodstream and therefore is protective of bone tissue.

Q: How much sleep do I need?
A: At least 6 to 8 hours a night. Quality sleep is foremost, which means it's better to have one eight-hour regulated period each night than several naps spaced out over the course of the day. As you get older your body requires less sleep, but not lesser quality sleep. If you have a chronic problem with waking and being unable to fall back to sleep, don't just lie there tossing and turning—get up and do something. Even walking around the house until you're fatigued is better than lying there.

Don't nap during the day—it will affect your sleep at night. And above all, don't take sleeping pills—they are highly addictive. Over-the-counter medications have benadryl, an antihistamine, in them, which acts as a hypnotic. It can leave you with a hangover the following day and promote poor sleep the next night.

Q: Why do the elderly typically sleep so poorly?
A: Older people tend to have more free time and a flexible schedule, so they may nap frequently during the day and therefore not be tired at night. They may suffer from urinary incontinence or prostate problems that can wake them from a sound sleep to use the bathroom. Insomnia may also result from worrying. A negative mental attitude can affect the quality and quantity of sleep.

Patients always report that they're sleeping better when they eat right and get lots of exercise. If you're really physically tired, your body will welcome a chance to relax completely.

Q: Will a small "toddy" before bedtime help to induce sleep?
A: One big myth is that a drink before bed will send you off to sleep. The truth is that alcohol is not a sleep inducer at all—it actually causes a disturbance in the quality of sleep and prevents the sleeper from getting down to the deepest stage of non-REM sleep that promotes a fine, rested feeling the next morning.

Q: Will exercise make me live longer?
A: Exercise alone doesn't guarantee longevity. The scientific literature suggests that you may live a year or a year and a half longer if you walk ten miles a week or the equivalent in some other form of exercise. But that's like saying you only lose 100 calories if you jog a mile. You're not doing exercise for the short-term results. The long-term benefits are definitely worth it. If you exercise regularly, the quality of your life will improve because you'll simply feel better about yourself. Exercise also makes you more resistant to disease. In the Framingham Heart Study, 17,000 Harvard alumni were surveyed on their exercise habits. Those who exercised and burned in excess of 2,000 calories a week (walking approximately three miles a day, every day) had a 28 percent lower risk of suffering a fatal coronary attack. Statistically, half of those people who have a heart attack have a massive one and die; the other 50 percent live. Exercise will allow you to be more functional for a longer period of time as you age.

Q: Does the Anti-Aging Diet prevent cancer?

A: No, nor does it treat cancer. Many cancers are caused by environmental factors—these are difficult if not impossible for us to avoid. Rose Fritch, a researcher in the Department of Epidemiology at Harvard Medical School, did a study that strongly indicated that college athletes had less incidence of cancer of the uterus, ovaries, and breast. After they graduated, those athletes who continued to exercise also continued to lower their risk.

Diet is also a significant protective factor. Civilizations with higher fiber diets have a lower incidence of cancer of the colon, prostate, breast, and uterus.

Skin cancer is directly related to sun exposure. If you stay out of the sun, you have only a 1 percent chance of contracting skin cancer.

Bone cancer appears to be environmentally stimulated. The majority of bone cancers occur secondary to other cancers like those of the lung, liver, or prostate.

Unfortunately, cancer is a complex disease involving a multitude of factors. But exercise, diet, an avoidance of environmental hazards, and positive mental attitude are all important in our self-immunization against cancer.

Q: My hands and feet seem colder in general than they used to be. Could this be a sign of aging?

A: There's no well-defined reason for this common complaint. Some possible causes include circulatory deficiency or a low thyroid function. However, the reason for this condition is seldom easily diagnosed. As you age, your metabolic rate slows down, which may also cause your body to feel colder.

Q: How do I know whether a symptom is really serious and if I should see a doctor?

A: You don't know if a symptom is serious. However, if you simply don't feel as well as you have in the past or feel totally different from your norm, you may need professional advice. Many diseases often cause you to simply feel different and may have only one minor symptom if any in the early stages.

If in doubt, see your doctor and be evaluated.

Q: Does it matter where I live as I age?
A: Warmer climates are more conducive to outdoor living. Therefore living in the South and the Southwest, where you can be involved in your community, can be healing physically and emotionally. I feel that the Sun Belt is generally a healthier place to live.

Q: Do our bodies get less flexible as we age?
A: Yes, but only because most people tend not to work on their flexibility by bending and stretching. Eastern philosophy says that a supple spine is the key to longevity, and healthful practices such as yoga and tai ch'i are part of daily life.
Gentle bending and stretching when you get out of bed in the morning every day will keep you flexible.

Q: Is it more difficult for my body to tolerate alcohol the older I get?
A: Yes. I feel you should drink less alcohol as you age, certainly no more than several ounces a week. The reason is that any drug or medication consumed by an elderly person is going to be absorbed much differently than if it were taken by a younger person— and drug dosages are generally minimized when prescribed for an older person, for just this reason. Consequently, since alcohol is a drug, I suggest that the older you get, the more cautious you should be about alcohol consumption. Also, the combined effect of alcohol with any medication is even more dangerous in an older person than a younger one. In addition, alcohol has a cumulative effect on the liver; the damage doesn't occur all at once. Alcoholic cirrhosis is a result of years of constant drinking and can strike hard in the elderly.

Q: Will I get shorter as I age?
A: There's no question about it—we all lose a certain amount of height because the vertebral bodies compress as we age. It's also possible to shrink one to two inches because the disk spaces between the vertebrae degenerate. In addition, in osteoporosis, the demineralization of bone that has become so common in the el-

derly in our society may cause a further loss of height. This makes the body hunch over and appear shorter as well.

Q: Will my breasts inevitably start to sag as I get older? What can I do to keep them from sagging? Will weight lifting or isometrics help?

A: Breast tissue is composed of fatty tissue and connective tissue that is affected by gravity. As connective tissue loses its elasticity over the years, breasts tend to sag, particularly in women who are overweight. Large breasts tend to become pendulous. There's not a great deal you can do to counteract the effects of gravity over the years. But weight lifting will strengthen and tone the underlying muscles of the breasts, giving them an enhanced appearance. Your breasts can look better at fifty than they did at twenty, particularly if you're not overly well endowed.

Q: I weigh the same as I did in college but my body weight seems to have shifted. I look fatter and my clothes don't fit as well. Why does this happen and what can I do about it?

A: Although you may weigh the same as you did in college, if you haven't exercised in a while, your body weight has probably shifted to the places where you'd prefer it not to. Your waist is probably thicker and your hips, buttocks, and thighs have probably increased in size. The good news is that all of this can change when you start a daily aerobic exercise program that will facilitate the burning of fat tissue in your problem areas. Your clothes can and will fit again!

Q: Some say we mellow as we age; others say we get old and crotchety and intolerant of change. Why is this? Can we do anything that will make us age well and wisely emotionally?

A: Someone once suggested that Ralph Nader was mellowing. He took this to mean that he had lost his bite, and his reply was that he certainly hoped he hadn't because it was a sure sign of aging. But mellowing doesn't have to mean "softening." You can still be outspoken and opinionated but perhaps with a more philosophical bent as you age. Older people who seem to be intolerant and divisive aren't happy people, but they probably weren't contented with their lives when they were younger, either. Your enthusiasm for life can continue indefinitely if you want it to and if you maintain a positive mental attitude. I've met people in their nineties who seem to have kept the same vigor they had in their youth.

What can we do to stay vital and mentally alert, not soft? Exercise is one of the best ways to give you a more positive approach to life. This doesn't mean that it will make you see the world through rose-colored glasses, only that you'll be able to use your lifetime's experience to understand that things can always change for the better.

Q: Is the older brain capable of learning new things? Can you really master Chinese or computers in your eighties? How do brain-retention changes affect you as you age?

A: My experience with my patients is that those who continue to read and study well into their eighties and nineties are the ones who maintain the highest level of mental acuity. They seem to remember things much better and continue to function mentally and emotionally better as they age than their peers. I think the combination of a mind stimulated by reading about something that interests you and a body exercised to keep your brain and nervous system fit is the best combination of elements to promote learning throughout life.

Q: Will my digestive system change as I age? How do I know if my new elimination habits are normal or not?

A: The digestive system slows down as we age, and it's for this reason that constipation can be a problem in elderly people. Some people may have a daily bowel movement; others may not have one for a week. There's no cause for concern unless the changes you see differ greatly from your previous norm. You must consult your physician concerning any dramatic changes in your overall bowel habits. Remember, though, that increasing the amount of fiber you eat, as you will be on the Anti-Aging Diet, as well as exercising daily will help you to improve and regulate your bowel habits.

Q: **What causes male and female incontinence? Whenever I see ads for adults' diapers on TV I get worried that it's going to happen to me someday. What can I do to prevent it?**
A: Urinary incontinence doesn't have to be part of your future. Often, this is a secondary response to medications that may not allow the body to control the urinary function. True incontinence can be surgically corrected, but the best advice is to maintain your overall health so that medication will not be necessary.

Q: **How long can my teeth last? How about my gums? How much dental health is genetic and how much is based on good dental care?**
A: Some people have excellent teeth and gums and will never develop periodontal disease. Use of alcohol and tobacco seem to be contributory factors that may lead to periodontal disease as you get older, so if you smoke and drink, I advise you to stop. You should also have regular dental checkups and cleanings twice a year.

Q: **Until what age can I drive a car? Will I necessarily have impaired night vision as I get older?**
A: Some people can drive a car well into their nineties. Generally, corrective lenses are all you need to improve problems you're having with your vision. Be sure to see your optometrist once a year to have your eyes checked.

Q: **Is it true that your foot size changes with age? How should I take care of my feet as I age?**
A: Generally, foot changes can occur as you age, and the changes are usually due to minor deformities such as bunions or flat feet. Whatever changes occur shouldn't be dramatic and certainly shouldn't concern you. Wear proper shoes, especially when exercising.

Q: **Does our perception of time stretch or collapse as we age? Older people say things like, "It seems like only yesterday" for long-distant events but they can't remember where they parked** the car at the mall. Why is this? Is there a difference in short-term and long-term memory loss?

A: Some people will develop memory loss as they age. The question is whether this loss is due to the normal aging process or whether it may be a sign of a more serious and progressive situation, such as Alzheimer's disease. It's very common not to remember the name or phone number of someone you met yesterday—not just for elderly people but for younger people as well. Short-term memory is designed to help you keep your place just as long as you need the information, like where you parked your car. Long-term memory, however, which includes the knowledge of a foreign language as well as the experience of a childhood birthday party, seems to improve with age.

Again, one of the best ways to maintain your mental acuity as you age is not just to read but also to exercise on a regular basis.

Q: As I get older, am I more likely to suffer injuries, like falling down, tripping, burning myself? Why?

A: No, not really. This all depends on how careful you are. Although elderly people appear to be more prone to falling, this is not an inevitable occurrence. Exercising will keep you balanced and agile and your muscles toned and strengthened. Medications can also affect your balance by causing dizziness and fainting.

Q: Does it take long for an injury to heal when you're older? How much longer and why?

A: It's true that your body does not respond as well to injuries at 85 as it does at 25. However, by maintaining proper nutrition and strengthening your immune system and your own self-healing capabilities, you'll be surprised how much more quickly your body can snap back.

Q: What's the top age of marathon runners? Will I have to change my type of exercise if I'm a real gung-ho exercise addict in my thirties?

A: One of the best-known marathon runners is John Kelly, with whom I had the pleasure of running in the 1978 Boston Marathon. John Kelly is now well into his eighties and runs the Boston Marathon in approximately five hours. Most scientific research suggests that people who exercise when they're younger may continue to exercise when they're older without any evidence of an increased formation of arthritis or other musculoskeletal injuries. This would include any knee, hip, or foot problems.

Q: How much damage can I undo if I never exercised or ate right before? How long will it take?

A: Your body will respond amazingly well to exercise, regardless of how inactive you've previously been. In just about thirty days, exercising every day, you can increase your aerobic capacity by 50 percent and your strength by almost 100 percent. Furthermore, lowering your protein consumption can help to facilitate a decrease in your blood cholesterol level by as much as 50 percent in only thirty days. The bottom line is that it's never too late to start exercising and eating properly.

Q: At my lunch break, I generally go out to delis and lunch-eonettes with office colleagues. What food choices are the least of all evils?

A: I suggest you order soup, bread, salad with dressing on the side, and a fruit plate. Almost all delis have these foods on the menu.

Q: I see all these "lite" products in the supermarket. How much less fat is there really? Can I eat some "lite" cheese and ice cream without going over my fat limit for the day?

A: My suggestion is that you avoid most of these "lite" products. The Anti-Aging Diet will get you back to the basics, which are not only less expensive but also lower in fat and lower in calories on a long-term basis. Many of these products marked "lite" are rather deceptive. Please read labels carefully! Make sure you know what's in the products marked "lite," "natural," "low in salt," or "low in calories."

Q: My family refuses to cut out meat. How can I stick to the Anti-Aging Diet when I have to prepare meat for everyone else?

A: It's usually impossible to change yourself or your family overnight to a mainly vegetarian diet. You have to do it gradually, introducing new foods and cutting out old ones over a long period of time. I think the recipes in this book are tempting enough to get even a diehard meat-eater interested, particularly because meats, fish, and chicken are used as ingredients in so many of them. You may be surprised to see how quickly your family wants to experiment with eating better. And if you have it once or twice a week, a meat meal won't kill you—just make sure you keep the portions small.

Q: I've always been in the habit of preparing quick lunches—sandwiches or hot dogs. Is it okay to switch to turkey bologna and turkey hot dogs? I know they're loaded with sodium, but turkey's better than pork, right?
A: Both turkey and pork are high in fat and protein. I'd suggest that any animal protein—pork, beef, veal, lamb, turkey, or chicken—be consumed in moderation. And deli meats and any other prepared meats should be eaten the least often.

Q: Can't I get enough vitamins and minerals to extend my life span in the food I eat without taking supplements?
A: Although vitamin C and beta carotene can be obtained in most of the foods we eat, the quantity of vitamin E required to satisfy the body's antioxidant, anti-aging needs may be more difficult to obtain from food sources. Selenium is present in minimal quantity in most foods, therefore supplementation of vitamin E with selenium is recommended.

Q: Why does food affect aging so much?
A: Your body needs the food you consume for energy. However, excess food, particularly excess protein, must be assimilated and digested and processed by your liver, kidneys, heart, and other organs. This is extremely stressful on the body and causes premature degeneration of these organs, making them far older than your chronological age.

Q: Does the Anti-Aging Diet require a lot of time and money?
A: The Anti-Aging Diet is easier than any other diet you've

ever been on. It doesn't require cooking special meals or purchasing special costly foods. In fact, it's actually less expensive than any other diet because you're eliminating high-cost foods such as veal, pork, ham, steak, ribs, and other sources of animal protein.

Most salads, fruits, vegetables, legumes, and grains—the staples of this diet—are very low cost items. You'll be delighted to see the difference in your supermarket cash register receipts each week.

Q: How does my self-esteem affect aging?

A: If your self-esteem is low, you will age quickly. Take for example the 65-year-old executive who retires and immediately loses the network of support he got from having a career. No one is praising his work any more, and he has no employees taking directions from him on a daily basis. Unless this man has other support systems in place to maintain his energy drive and enthusiasm for living, he will undoubtedly age quickly.

Self-image is extremely important in determining how old you think you are. Negative thought, fear, jealousy, hatred, and despair are all qualities that appear on your face and in your body, aging your appearance, and wearing you down emotionally as well.

Q: Would you consider the Japanese diet as healthy as the Anti-Aging Diet?

A: A century ago, I would have said that the Japanese ate the healthiest diet on earth, although people certainly didn't live as long because they succumbed to a variety of diseases. But the diet was extremely healthy—meat was used only as a condiment or side dish and therefore the amount of animal protein consumed was minimal.

Today, however, beef consumption has soared in Japan as has the use of dairy products, including ice cream. The Japanese have not only adopted our American high-fat, high-protein diet but also our propensity for heart disease, strokes, and stomach cancer.

For these reasons, it's clear that the Anti-Aging Diet is far healthier than the diet of 1990s Japan.

Q: Is a vegetarian diet the ultimate diet?

A: A vegetarian, low-protein diet is certainly a healthful diet choice. The complete elimination of animal products in combination with a well-balanced diet of plant-based foods will give you an additional edge on longevity. But for those long accustomed to animal products, for whom eliminating all meat, fish, cheese, and so on would be a real hardship and impossible to comply with over the long run, the Anti-Aging Diet is the ultimate diet.

Q: Is old age a cause of death?
A: No. Aging is a developmental process that begins the day we're born. Advanced age brings with it a variety of physical changes, but in the absence of disease, none of these changes are killers. A person who has followed good nutrition and exercise habits from an early age is going to have more stamina, energy, strength, and agility in extreme old age than one who hasn't.

Part Four

Recipes

When I decided to contact some of the leading restaurants in Phoenix to create recipes for the Anti-Aging Diet, I wasn't sure whether the chefs would want to participate. After all, steaks, chops, eggs, and all those animal-based protein foods are the staples of any restaurant menu.

I was therefore happily surprised at the overwhelming response I received from some of the very finest culinary hot spots. Their chefs came up with dozens of delectable recipes that went right along with my anti-aging menu plan.

Several of these chefs—Chris Bianco of Bianco's, Vincent Guerithault of Vincent's on Camelback, Benito Mellino of Avanti's, and Christopher Gross of Christopher's—all confided to me that these new recipes have become the most popular on their own menus and that their patrons specifically ask for "anti-aging" foods when they come in. One of the best comments I've heard is that none of our extraordinary recipes taste remotely as though they belong on a diet.

Although there are plenty of recipe selections for the all-American palate, quite naturally we rely pretty heavily on the wonderfully low-protein foods of the Southwest—recipes based on beans, corn, and interesting chilis. I've also included many of my favorites from different Asian cuisines—Chinese and Thai, specifically—because these recipes come from traditions in which meats are used as condiments and for flavoring and in which vegetables and grains are the primary ingredients.

You'll note that our recipe headings are different from those in many other cookbooks or diet books. Our main dishes are hearty soups, stews, salads, legumes, and grain dishes. When eaten as main courses, with your chicken, beef, or fish accompaniment, with a whole grain bread (unbuttered!) on the side and fruit for dessert, they provide an exciting, low-protein meal that is as appropriate for an elegant dinner party as it is for a daily family spread.

A word about salt: Sodium is an essential nutrient, and we all need it to survive. The minimum daily requirement of daily salt intake, however, is only ¼ teaspoon—a great deal less than most people consume. It's not necessary to add any salt at all to our recipes, because sodium is a natural constituent of most if not all the foods in each recipe. However, if you are currently a high-salt user, it will take you some time to reprogram your taste buds. You may either add a *small* amount of salt to each recipe, or you may add a few grains at the table (after you've tasted the food, of course!).

In Chapter 5 (pages 67–130) are four one-week sample menus— one each at 50, 60, 75, and 85 grams of protein. These will serve as guidelines for the Anti-Aging Diet. Putting it simply, you will be limiting all foods of animal origin and eating abundantly from foods of plant origin. Naturally, you'll be adjusting the servings depending on where you are in the diet.

When you're on the first stage of the Anti-Aging Diet—weight loss—the percentage of daily protein will be about 20 percent of your daily caloric intake.

When you are within five pounds of your goal weight and proceed to the lifetime program, the second stage (pages 117–130), you may have unlimited servings of fruits, vegetables, grains, and most legumes, but your animal protein intake will not change. This means that as you increase calories to maintain your new slim weight, the percentage of protein you're eating will actually decrease to a healthier lifetime range of about 10 percent of your total daily caloric intake.

I've included information about calories, fat, and sodium for those of you on any restricted diets. The sample menu plans, creative menu planners, and protein-gram counters in Chapter 5 will be your guide to help you control portion sizes of high-protein foods.

The great variety of meal choices is intended to offer you many opportunities to mix and match tastes at your table. You may substitute one similar food for another, or you may repeat meals or days, as you desire.

Remember that the success of this new style of eating depends on you. Be brave enough to try new tastes, but don't exclude the old ones you love. No food group is eliminated on the Anti-Aging Diet, which means that you have a wide range of foods in each food group to choose from that offers both the key to long-term successful weight management as well as the bonus of anti-aging benefits.

Enjoy! It's time to learn to eat in a healthful way that will not only take off unwanted pounds, but will enhance your potential for growing younger as the years pass.

Chapter 12

Appetizers and Accompaniments

Red and Yellow Bell Pepper Soup

This is actually a colorful blend of two soups and would create the perfect party atmosphere when used as an appetizer for Grilled Shrimp Salad with Frizzled Tortillas (see page 230).

RED PEPPER SOUP

- 2 large red bell peppers
- 1 tablespoon olive oil
- 1 tablespoon chopped shallots

- 2 cups defatted chicken stock
- 1 cup nonfat plain yogurt Freshly ground black pepper

YELLOW PEPPER SOUP

- 2 large yellow bell peppers
- 1 tablespoon olive oil
- 1 tablespoon chopped shallots

- 2 cups defatted chicken stock
- 1 cup nonfat plain yogurt Freshly ground black pepper

1. Preheat oven to 250°F.

2. Place both the red and yellow peppers on a cookie sheet and roast for about 10 minutes. Peel the peppers and dice them but do not mix the colors. Set aside.

3. *For Red Pepper Soup:* In a medium saucepan, heat the olive oil and sauté the shallots for about 1 minute over low heat. Then add the red peppers and sauté for about 2 minutes more. Stir in the chicken stock and cook for 10 minutes over low heat. Stir in the yogurt during the last minute but do not allow to come to a boil. Add freshly ground black pepper to taste. Put the mixture into a blender and blend until smooth. Return to the saucepan to keep warm while making Yellow Pepper Soup.

4. *For Yellow Pepper Soup:* In a medium saucepan, heat the olive oil and sauté the shallots for about 1 minute over low heat. Then add the yellow peppers and sauté for about 2 minutes more. Stir in the chicken stock and cook for 10 minutes over low heat. Stir in the yogurt during the last minute but do not allow to come to a boil. Add freshly ground black pepper to taste. Put the mixture into a blender and blend until smooth. Return to the saucepan and keep warm until ready to serve.

5. To serve, use two ladles and slowly pour the two soups simultaneously into the soup bowls, one color on each side. Serve hot.

Yields: 8 servings
Serving size: about 1 cup
Calories per serving: 118

Grams of protein per serving: 5
Grams of fat per serving: 4
Milligrams of sodium per serving: 254

Recipe courtesy of Vincent Guerithault of Vincent's on Camelback.

Marinated Mandarin Shrimp

Here's an appetizer whose refreshing combination of flavors will have guests calling for the recipe.

2 11-ounce cans mandarin orange segments in light syrup
½ cup thinly sliced small white onions

½ cup thinly sliced red or green bell pepper
2 pounds cooked, shelled, and deveined shrimp, fresh or frozen

MARINADE:

2 tablespoons sugar
1 teaspoon salt (optional)
1 teaspoon freshly ground black pepper
1 tablespoon mustard seed or powder
½ tablespoon celery seed
¼ teaspoon dried hot red peppers

2 tablespoons chopped parsley
2 cloves garlic, crushed
¾ cup rice vinegar* or any mild vinegar
¼ cup vegetable oil
¼ cup water
⅓ cup fresh lemon or lime juice
¼ cup ketchup

1. Drain the oranges. Place the oranges, onions, peppers, and shrimp in a shallow, 2-quart glass bowl.
2. Combine all the marinade ingredients. Stir to mix thoroughly and pour over the shrimp mixture. Cover and refrigerate, allowing the mixture to marinate for at least 24 hours.
3. Serve in marinade with toothpicks.

Yields: 12 servings
Serving size: about ½ cup
Calories per serving: 145
Grams of protein per serving: 14

Grams of fat per serving: 5
Milligrams of sodium per serving: 133
(300 if optional salt is added)

Recipe courtesy of Southwest Health Institute.

*Rice vinegar is available in Oriental markets or the ethnic section of your supermarket.

Jalapeño-Honey Cornbread

This bread is a nice complement for a soup or salad.

¾ cup cornmeal	2 tablespoons honey
½ cup whole wheat flour	2 cups crushed cooked corn
½ cup all-purpose flour	2 tablespoons chopped
1 teaspoon baking soda	canned jalapeño peppers
1 whole egg or 2 egg whites	tablespoons vegetable oil
1 cup buttermilk	

1. Preheat oven to 400°F. Lightly oil a 9-inch-square baking dish.
2. Mix together all the dry ingredients and set aside.
3. In another bowl, beat the egg with a fork. Stir in the remaining ingredients.
4. Combine the dry and liquid ingredients, mixing only until all dry ingredients are moistened. Do not overmix. Pour the batter into the prepared baking dish and bake for approximately 20 minutes or until a toothpick inserted into the center comes out clean.

Yields: 9-inch-square loaf   *Grams of protein per serving: 4*
Serving size: 3-inch square   *Grams of fat per serving: 4*
Calories per serving: 144   *Milligrams of sodium per serving: 156*

Recipe courtesy of Southwest Health Institute.

Fresh Salsa

Serve as a dip, a salad dressing, topping for baked potatoes, and as a condiment with all Mexican recipes.

1 fresh green chili (if you want a hotter sauce, use 2)	½ teaspoon fresh cilantro or a pinch of dried
2 fresh ripe tomatoes (about 1 pound), chopped	½ teaspoon ground cumin
2 cloves garlic, minced	1 tablespoon unsalted tomato sauce
4 green onions, tops and bulbs, chopped	1 tablespoon fresh lime juice
	½ teaspoon salt, optional

1. Preheat oven to 350°F.
2. Wash the green chili but do not cut it. Place the whole chili on a cookie sheet and roast for about 15 minutes or until the chili begins to soften. Remove it from the oven, cool, and dice the chili. Discard the seeds.
3. Combine all the ingredients in a food processor or blender. Process or blend just until all ingredients are finely chopped. Do not puree.
4. Chill and serve.

Yields: 2 cups
Serving size: 1/4 cup
Calories per serving: 20

Grams of protein per serving: 1
Grams of fat per serving: 0
Milligrams of sodium per serving: 165

Recipe courtesy of Southwest Health Institute.

Salsa Pronto

This salsa utilizes the convenience of shelf-ready products. Use it when time is limited or if the condition of fresh tomatoes is less than desirable.

Serve it as you would the fresh salsa. This salsa keeps for several weeks in a covered jar in the refrigerator.

1 16-ounce can peeled unsalted tomatoes, drained
1 4-ounce can peeled mild green chilies, chopped
4 green onions, bulbs and tops, chopped
3 cloves garlic, minced
1 tablespoon unsalted tomato paste
1 tablespoon fresh lime juice
1/4 teaspoon chili powder
1/4 teaspoon ground cumin
Pinch of cilantro
Salt to taste

1. Combine all the ingredients in a food processor or blender. Process or blend only until all the ingredients are finely chopped. Do not puree.
2. Chill and serve.

Yields: 2 cups
Serving size: ¼ cup
Calories per serving: 22

Grams of protein per serving: 1
Grams of fat per serving: 0
Milligrams of sodium per serving: 176

Vegetable Stock

Many of our recipes call for either chicken or vegetable stock. Here is a versatile vegetable stock recipe that can be made in quantity and frozen for later use.

1 leek, cleaned and coarsely chopped
2 medium onions, coarsely chopped
2 medium carrots, coarsely chopped
2 medium parsnips, peeled and coarsely chopped
2 celery stalks, coarsely chopped

2 large tomatoes, coarsely chopped
2 cloves garlic, crushed
1 small bunch cilantro, fresh snipped
1 teaspoon whole black peppercorns
Salt to taste
10 cups cold water

1. Place all the ingredients in a large stockpot. Bring to a boil over high heat, then reduce heat and simmer about 1 hour, uncovered.

2. Strain. Use immediately or cool and freeze for later use.

Yields: about 6 cups
Serving size: 1 cup
Calories per serving: 65

Grams of protein per serving: 2
Grams of fat per serving: 0
Milligrams of sodium per serving: 35

Recipe courtesy of Christopher Gross of Christopher's.

Hot Mustard Dip

This dip is especially good with crisp, raw jicama* but is fine with any raw vegetables.

2 eggs, well beaten
½ cup sugar
2 tablespoons dry mustard

½ cup water
1 cup apple cider

1. Combine all the ingredients in a small saucepan and stir over low heat until the mixture is slightly thickened.
2. Cool and serve.

Yields: 2 cups
Serving size: 2 tablespoons
Calories per serving: 42

Grams of protein per serving: 1
Grams of fat per serving: 1
Milligrams of sodium per serving: 8

Recipe courtesy of Southwest Health Institute.
*Jicama is available in Spanish bodegas or supermarkets.

Vegetable "Tea"

2 tomatoes, halved and seeded
7 medium carrots, chopped
2 medium onions, sliced
½ medium leek, cleaned and chopped
1 stalk celery
½ bay leaf, broken up

1 sprig fresh parsley
1 sprig fresh thyme
1 sprig fresh tarragon
2 cloves garlic
2 shallots, sliced
Pinch of freshly ground black pepper

1. Place all the ingredients in a 2-quart canning jar. Fill to ¾ inch from the top with water and cover with lid. Cook in a water bath for 2½ hours.
2. Remove the jar from the water bath and let cool before opening because the "tea" will be under pressure. When cool, open and strain.

3. Use hot or cold, as a soup stock, a seasoning for cooked vegetables, or in recipes calling for vegetable stock. Freezes well.

Yields: about 6 cups   *Grams of protein per serving: 2*
Serving size: 1 cup   *Grams of fat per serving: 0*
Calories per serving: 71   *Milligrams of sodium per serving: 43*

Recipe courtesy of Chris Bianco of Bianco's.

Chapter 13

Main Dish Salads

Neapolitan Potato Salad

Wonderful for picnics and warm summer days, served with a big green salad—but just as good in the winter with a chicken or fish dish by its side.

6 large potatoes (about
1½ pounds)
1 medium onion, chopped
2 tablespoons chopped fresh dill
2 tablespoons chopped cilantro

1 tablespoon capers, rinsed
2 cloves garlic, minced
¼ cup extra-virgin light olive oil
Juice of 1 lemon
Salt and freshly ground black pepper

1. Scrub the potatoes well. Halve the potatoes horizontally and place them in a saucepan. Cover them with water and boil over medium-high heat until tender, about 40 minutes. Remove the potatoes from the water and allow them to cool.

2. Meanwhile, mix together the remaining ingredients, except the salt and pepper, and set aside.

3. After the potatoes have cooled, cut them into 1-inch slices and arrange the slices on a platter. Pour the olive oil mixture over the potatoes. Add salt and freshly ground black pepper to taste. Serve at room temperature.

Yields: 6 servings	*Grams of protein per serving: 4*
Serving size: about 1 cup	*Grams of fat per serving: 9*
Calories per serving: 183	*Milligrams of sodium per serving: 19*

Recipe courtesy of Benito of Avanti.

Grilled Chicken Caesar Salad

Caesar salad is traditionally off most diets but not the Anti-Aging Diet! The light dressing and skinless chicken make it a perfect low-protein meal.

1 head romaine lettuce, washed and well dried	2 4-ounce boneless chicken breasts, skin and all visible fat removed

DRESSING:

2 tablespoons extra-virgin light olive oil	10–12 drops Worcestershire sauce
2 pasteurized egg whites (Egg Beaters™ or any other brand)	1 clove garlic, squeezed through garlic press
1 teaspoon Dijon mustard	1 teaspoon dried tarragon
½ lemon	

TOPPING:

2 tablespoons grated Parmesan	Freshly ground black pepper
¼ cup croutons	

1. Break up the lettuce into large pieces and place in a large salad bowl.

2. Grill the chicken breasts for about 8 minutes on each side. Slice and keep warm.

3. Mix together the dressing ingredients and toss with the lettuce until the lettuce is well coated.

4. Divide the lettuce into 4 equal servings and place on individual serving plates. Top each serving with a quarter of the warm chicken slices. Evenly divide the Parmesan and croutons and sprinkle over each salad and serve.

> Yields: 4 salads
> Serving size: 2 ounces
> chicken per salad
> Calories per serving: 190
>
> Grams of protein per serving: 20
> Grams of fat per serving: 9
> Milligrams of sodium per serving: 157

Recipe courtesy of Benito of Avanti's.

Grilled Shrimp Salad with Frizzled Tortillas

2 6-inch blue corn tortillas
2 6-inch yellow corn tortillas
1/2 cup olive oil
1 tablespoon diced red bell pepper
1 tablespoon diced green bell pepper
1 tablespoon diced yellow bell pepper
1 tablespoon julienned fresh ginger
2 tablespoons chopped fresh basil

2 tablespoons sherry wine vinegar
Salt and freshly ground black pepper
1 tablespoon diced tomato
About 10 cups assorted greens (lamb lettuce, red oak leaf lettuce, arugula, watercress), washed, drained, and torn
1 pound fresh shrimp, shelled and deveined

1. Put the blue and yellow corn tortillas through a pasta machine to make thin julienne strips or cut them with a knife into thin,

even, julienne strips. Heat the olive oil in a skillet and sauté the tortilla strips in olive oil over medium-high heat until crisp, about 5 minutes. When crisp, drain them thoroughly. Reserve 2 tablespoons of the warm olive oil to cook the shrimp and the rest for the dressing.

2. In a large salad bowl, combine the bell peppers, the ginger, the basil, the sherry wine vinegar, and all but 2 tablespoons of the warm olive oil. Toss the ingredients and add salt and freshly ground black pepper to taste. Add the tortilla strips and the assorted greens. Gently toss until mixed and divide into 4 equal servings. Place each serving on a separate plate.

3. Brush the shrimp lightly with the remaining 2 tablespoons of olive oil and grill them over a very hot fire for approximately 1 minute. Be careful not to overcook. Serve the hot shrimp on top of the salad.

Yields: 4 servings　　　　*Grams of protein per serving: 29*
Serving size: 4 ounces shrimp　*Grams of fat per serving: 30*
Calories per serving: 442　　*Milligrams of sodium per serving: 242*

Recipe courtesy of Vincent Guerithault of Vincent's on Camelback.

Oriental Cabbage Salad

4 cups shredded cabbage (1 small head)
½ cup thin strips green onions
⅓ cup rice vinegar* or any mild vinegar

Juice of 1 lemon
2 tablespoons reduced-sodium soy sauce
2 teaspoons sugar
Greens

1. In a large steamer, steam the shredded cabbage for 7 minutes, or until just barely tender. Or microwave in a 2-quart glass bowl with 2 tablespoons of water for 5 minutes, or until just barely tender.

2. Combine the cabbage and green onions in a 2-quart shallow dish.

3. In a bowl, stir together the remaining ingredients and pour over the cabbage and onions. Marinate for several hours.

4. To serve, arrange on a bed of greens.

Yields: 2 cups	Grams of protein per serving: 2
Serving size: ½ cup	Grams of fat per serving: 0
Calories per serving: 34	Milligrams of sodium per serving: 300

Recipe courtesy of Southwest Health Institute.

*Rice vinegar is available in Oriental markets or the ethnic section of your supermarket.

Sesame Pasta Salad

¾ pound angel hair pasta
3 cups thin strips cabbage
2 cups thinly sliced unpeeled cucumber
½ cup frozen green peas

1 cup julienne-cut green onions, bulbs and tops
6 ounces turkey ham or roast turkey breast
1 egg

DRESSING:

½ cup rice vinegar* or any mild vinegar
2 tablespoons water
⅓ cup sugar

1½ tablespoons canola oil
1½ tablespoons sesame oil
1 tablespoon sesame seeds

1. Prepare the pasta according to package directions. During the last minute of cooking, add the sliced cabbage. Do not overcook. Drain both the pasta and cabbage in a colander. Run cold water over both and let drain. Set aside with the remaining vegetables.

2. Slice the ham into thin slivers and reserve. Boil the egg until hard boiled, then cool by placing it in cold water. Peel the egg, slice it thinly, and reserve.

3. In a glass jar with a lid, mix together the dressing ingredients. Set aside.

4. In a large salad or serving bowl, toss together all the ingredients except the dressing. Shake the dressing, pour it over the salad, and mix thoroughly. Cover the salad and refrigerate for several hours.

5. Divide into 8 equal servings and place on individual plates. Serve.

Yields: 8 servings	Grams of protein per serving: 9
Serving size: about 2 cups	Grams of fat per serving: 8
Calories per serving: 186	Milligrams of sodium per serving: 130

Recipe courtesy of Southwest Health Institute.
*Rice vinegar is available in Oriental markets or the ethnic section of your supermarket.

Fennel and Watercress Salad with Blood Oranges and Pecans

Blood oranges, found in the south of Italy, give this salad a great burst of color and sunny flavor. But don't worry if you can't find them in the market; regular navel oranges work just as well.

1 bunch watercress, about 6 ounces
1 large fennel bulb, about 1 pound
2 large blood oranges or navel oranges

3 ounces pecans, coarsely chopped
Juice of 1 orange, any kind
1 tablespoon extra-virgin olive oil
Freshly ground black pepper

1. Trim about 1 inch off the bottom of the watercress to remove any fibrous or tough parts. Clean and trim the remaining watercress and place in a large bowl.

2. Cut off the top of the fennel bulb and remove the small tough core. Slice the bulb into the thinnest rings possible. Place the rings in the bowl with the watercress.

3. Peel and slice the oranges into rings and add to the bowl. Toast the chopped pecans by putting them on a cookie sheet in a preheated 350°F oven for 10 minutes. Add the toasted pecans.

4. In a separate bowl, whisk together the olive oil and orange juice. Pour the dressing over the salad and toss well.

5. To serve, add freshly ground black pepper to taste. Divide into 4 equal portions and place on individual serving plates.

Yields: 4 servings
Serving size: about 1 cup
Calories per serving: 241

Grams of protein per serving: 7
Grams of fat per serving: 17
Milligrams of sodium per serving: 28

Recipe courtesy of Chris Bianco of Bianco's.

Chapter 14

Legumes

Comilona (Bean-Feast) Dip

Serve this chilled as a dip with toasted corn tortillas or heated and spread on warmed corn or flour tortillas. This can also double as a quick microwave lunch with tortillas.

1 cup cooked pinto beans or canned vegetarian-style refried beans

¼ cup nonfat plain yogurt

¼ cup diced canned mild green chilies

1 teaspoon chili powder

1. Process cooked pinto beans in a food processor until a semismooth paste is formed. If using the canned refried beans, omit this step.

2. Combine all the ingredients in a small bowl and stir until blended.

3. Chill to use as a dip; warm to use as a spread.

Yields: 1½ cups dip
Serving size: ¼ cup
Calories per serving: 70

Grams of protein per serving: 4
Grams of fat per serving: 2
Milligrams of sodium per serving: 247

Recipe courtesy of Southwest Health Institute.

Black Bean Terrine with Goat Cheese

Serve this terrine with Fresh Salsa (page 223) or Marinated Carrots (page 252).

2 pounds dried black beans, rinsed and picked over
1 medium onion
1 carrot
1 fresh jalapeño pepper
4 eggs
2 tablespoons chopped fresh cilantro
Salt and freshly ground black pepper
1 tablespoon olive oil
8 ounces mild California goat cheese

1. In a large pot, soak the beans overnight in cold water to cover. Drain the beans, rinse, and pick over to remove any damaged beans. Return the beans to the pot and cover with 2 quarts of cold water. Add the onion, carrot, and chili. Cook over low heat for about 1 hour.

2. Drain the beans and discard the vegetables. Puree the beans in a food processor. Add the eggs and cilantro and freshly ground black pepper to taste. Process briefly to mix.

3. Preheat oven to 250°F.

4. Brush the sides of a 2–quart terrine with the olive oil and line it with parchment paper. Fill it with half of the bean puree, put the goat cheese in the center, and cover with the remainder of the bean puree.

5. Bake at 250°F in a bain marie for 1 hour. If you don't have a bain marie, set the terrine into a large baking pan and then add water until it's halfway up the terrine's sides and bake for 1 hour. Let cool and refrigerate overnight. Slice and serve cold with your favorite light sauce.

Yields: 8 servings
Serving size: 7 ounces
Calories per serving: 294
Grams of protein per serving: 13
Grams of fat per serving: 13
Milligrams of sodium per serving: 216

Recipe courtesy of Vincent Guerithault of Vincent's on Camelback.

Lentil and Brown Rice Soup

5 cups defatted chicken stock, or more as desired
3 cups water
1½ cups lentils, rinsed and picked over
1 cup brown rice
4 large tomatoes (about 1 pound), quartered
3 large carrots, halved lengthwise and cut into ¼-inch pieces
1 onion, chopped
3 stalks celery, chopped
3 cloves garlic, minced
1 teaspoon fresh or ½ teaspoon dried basil
½ teaspoon dried oregano
¼ teaspoon dried thyme
1 bay leaf
½ cup minced fresh parsley
2 tablespoons cider vinegar or lemon juice
Salt and freshly ground black pepper

1. In a large soup pot, combine all ingredients except the parsley, vinegar, salt, and pepper. Bring to a boil and simmer, covered, stirring occasionally, for 45 to 55 minutes, or until lentils and rice are cooked.

2. Stir in the parsley and vinegar or lemon juice. Season with salt and freshly ground black pepper to taste.

3. Soup will thicken as it stands. To serve, thin with additional chicken stock, if desired.

Yields: 8 servings
Serving size: about 1½ cups
Calories per serving: 274
Grams of protein per serving: 15
Grams of fat per serving: 2
Milligrams of sodium per serving: 202

Recipe courtesy of Benito of Avanti's.

Black Bean Cowboy Stew

1 pound dried black beans, rinsed and picked over	2 medium potatoes (about 4 ounces each), peeled and chopped
10 cups water	1 cup chopped onion
½ pound lean round or sirloin steak, coarsely chopped	½ cup chopped green bell pepper
1 1.8-ounce package Knorr Oxtail Soup and Recipe Mix	½ cup chopped red bell pepper
1 large carrot, chopped	Dash of Tabasco or other hot pepper sauce

1. Place the beans and the water in a large soup pot. Cover and soak overnight.

2. The next day, do not drain the beans. Stir in the meat and the soup mix. Simmer the mixture over low heat, covered, for 2 to 3 hours, stirring occasionally.

3. When the beans have begun to soften, add the remaining ingredients and continue to simmer over low heat, covered, for another hour, stirring occasionally.

4. Uncover the pot and allow to simmer, stirring occasionally, until the soup is thickened and all the vegetables are tender, about 30 minutes more. The time will depend on how finely you have chopped the vegetables.

Yields: About 12 cups
Serving size: 1 cup
Calories per serving: 216

Grams of protein per serving: 16
Grams of fat per serving: 3
Milligrams of sodium per serving: 353

Recipe courtesy of Southwest Health Institute.

Tortilla Pizza with Stir Fry Veggies and Black Bean Sauce

SAUCE:

2 cloves garlic, crushed
½ tablespoon olive oil
2 cups cooked or 1 15-ounce can vegetarian-style black beans

½ cup defatted chicken or vegetable stock

STIR FRY VEGETABLES:

1 tablespoon olive oil
2 medium green bell peppers, julienne sliced
1 small zucchini, julienne sliced
1 small yellow squash, julienne sliced

4 medium white mushrooms, julienne sliced
4 small plum tomatoes, seeded and chopped
Freshly ground black pepper, optional

TOPPING:

4 ounces mozzarella-style soya cheese, grated
2 green onions, bulbs and tops, chopped

4 sprigs fresh cilantro

2 large flour tortillas (about 11 inches)

1. *For sauce:* In a large skillet, sauté the garlic in the olive oil over medium heat until the garlic is light brown, about 3 minutes. Add the beans and stir. When warmed through, in about 5 minutes, add the stock, increase the heat to high, and bring to a boil. Then remove from the heat and puree in a food processor or blender until the mixture is smooth. (If a thicker consistency is desired,

just return the mixture to the pan until the mixture resembles a thick sauce.) Set aside until the assembly step.

2. *For stir fry vegetables:* Pour the olive oil into a large skillet. Add the vegetables and stir fry over medium heat about 5 or 10 minutes, or until softened. Season with freshly ground black pepper if desired. Set aside until the assembly step.

3. *Assembly:* Preheat the broiler for a few minutes. Place the tortillas on pizza pans or a cookie sheet and lightly toast both sides, about 1 minute each side. Remove from the oven and spread each tortilla with half the bean sauce. Then top each with half the vegetable mixture. Top each pizza with 2 ounces of the grated cheese and return to the broiler until the cheese is melted, about 5 minutes. Then decorate each with equal amounts of onion and cilantro.

Yields: 2 11-inch pizzas
Serving size: ½ pizza
Calories per serving: 343

Grams of protein per serving: 18
Grams of fat per serving: 12
Milligrams of sodium per serving: 302

Recipe courtesy of Chris Bianco of Bianco's.

Chapter 15

Main Dish Pasta, Potatoes, and Rice

Whole Wheat Pasta with Fresh Tomato and Basil Sauce

1 small white onion, chopped
2 tablespoons extra-virgin olive oil
1 pound plum tomatoes, chopped
3 cloves garlic, minced

2 sprigs fresh basil, chopped
Freshly ground black pepper
1 pound whole wheat spaghetti pasta (we recommend DiCecco)

TOPPING:

2 tablespoons grated Parmesan

2 sprigs basil, chopped

1. In a large pot, bring 6 quarts of water to a boil for cooking pasta.
2. Meanwhile, in a sauté pan, sauté the onion in the olive oil over medium-high heat until the onion is transparent, about 5 minutes. Add the chopped tomatoes, garlic, and basil. Continue to

cook over low heat until the tomatoes soften and the mixture is saucelike, about 20 minutes. Add freshly ground black pepper to taste. Keep warm.

3. Add the pasta to the boiling water and cook until tender. Drain.

4. To serve, divide the pasta into 6 equal servings and place each on a serving plate. Pour an equal amount of sauce on each serving and sprinkle with Parmesan cheese and fresh basil.

Yields: 6 servings	*Grams of protein per serving: 11*
Serving size: about 1½ cups	*Grams of fat per serving: 6*
pasta and ½ cup sauce	*Milligrams of sodium per serving: 9*
Calories per serving: 354	

Recipe courtesy of Benito of Avanti's.

Chef Vincent's Chipotle Pasta

Chipotle chili puree is imported from Mexico. If your gourmet store doesn't carry it, you can substitute a commercial Chinese bean paste. Just be careful with the amount if you're nervous about spices—select one marked mild or medium.

1 cup all-purpose flour	Salt
1 tablespoon chipotle chili	Salt and freshly ground
puree	black pepper
1 extra-large egg	Chopped fresh cilantro
1 teaspoon olive oil	

1. In a food processor, briefly process the flour with the Chipotle puree until mixed. Add the egg and process to mix. Add the olive oil and a dash of salt. Process until the mixture forms a small ball around the blade. It may be necessary to add 1 teaspoon of water.

2. Put dough through a pasta machine to desired size. If you have no pasta machine, roll out the pasta to ⅛-inch thickness. Cut into desired size. Hang on a rack to dry.

3. When ready to serve, cook the dried pasta in boiling salted

water for approximately 15 seconds. Drain. Season with salt and freshly ground black pepper to taste. Garnish with chopped cilantro and serve hot.

Yields: 2 servings
Serving size: 1½ cups pasta
Calories per serving: 287

Grams of protein per serving: 10
Grams of fat per serving: 6
Milligrams of sodium per serving: 31

Recipe courtesy of Vincent Guerithault of Vincent's on Camelback.

Zucchini-Mushroom Lasagne

1   12-ounce package lasagne
    noodles
1   cup part-skim ricotta
2   tablespoons skim milk
1   recipe of Marinara Sauce
    (page 246) or 3 cups
    marinara sauce

2   cups shredded zucchini
1   cup shiitake mushrooms,
    sliced
4   ounces part-skim
    mozzarella, grated
    Fresh parsley sprigs

1. Preheat oven to 350°F.
2. Cook lasagne noodles according to package directions. Drain and reserve.
3. Blend the ricotta and skim milk together in a blender until smooth.
4. Spread one third of the marinara sauce on the bottom and sides of a 9-inch-square baking dish. (Use a microwave-safe dish if you're going to microwave it.) Cover with half of the lasagne noodles, spread with half of the ricotta-milk mixture, sprinkle with half of the zucchini, half of the mushrooms, and half of the mozzarella. Repeat this procedure. Top with the remaining third of the marinara sauce.
5. Bake uncovered in the oven for approximately 30 minutes. This dish can also be covered and microwaved until heated through, about 10 minutes.

6. Cut into 3-inch squares to serve and garnish with fresh parsley sprigs.

> Yields: 9 servings
> Serving size: 1 3-inch square
> Calories per serving: 161
>
> Grams of protein per serving: 9
> Grams of fat per serving: 6
> Milligrams of sodium per serving: 106

Recipe courtesy of Southwest Health Institute.

Linguini with Broccoli Sauce

2 pounds fresh broccoli
¾ cup water from cooking broccoli
4 cloves garlic, minced
1 tablespoon olive oil
1 pound imported Italian linguini or other pasta

Juice of ½ lemon
Salt and freshly ground black pepper
2 tablespoons pine nuts (or grated Parmesan, optional)
1 teaspoon grated lemon peel

1. Bring a large pot of water to a boil. Clean the broccoli and slice it lengthwise. Blanch the broccoli in the boiling water about 7 to 10 minutes or until the hard stalks yield to the touch. Remove the broccoli and chop coarsely. Reserve about ¾ cup of the broccoli water.

2. In a large sauté pan or a wok, sauté the garlic in the olive oil over medium-high heat until light brown, about 5 minutes. Then add the chopped broccoli and sauté on medium heat for 5 minutes. Add the broccoli water, increase the heat, and cook until the liquid is reduced. Smash the broccoli with a wooden spoon until it is in a sauce form.

3. While the broccoli is cooking, cook the pasta according to package directions. Drain the pasta and mix with the broccoli sauce and lemon juice. Season with freshly ground black pepper to taste.

4. Toss the pine nuts in a skillet over high heat for 2 minutes to toast.

5. To serve, top with toasted pine nuts and grated lemon peel.

Yields: 6 servings
Serving size: 2 cups
Calories per serving: 331

Grams of protein per serving: 13
Grams of fat per serving: 5
Milligrams of sodium per serving: 40

Recipe courtesy of Chris Bianco of Bianco's.

Penne with Tomato, Basil, and Garlic Sauce

2 28-ounce cans imported
   Italian tomatoes
8 cloves garlic, minced
¼ teaspoon red pepper flakes

10 fresh basil leaves
1   pound imported Italian
    penne or other small pasta

1. Place the tomatoes in a large sauté pan, break them up, and bring to a boil over medium-high heat. Add the garlic and reduce the heat to medium. Stir in the red pepper flakes. Cook about 10 or 15 minutes or to desired thickness. Tear 8 of the basil leaves into small pieces and add them to the sauce when it is just about done. (This timing insures that the flavor and color of the basil will be retained.)

2. Cook the pasta according to package directions and drain. You may add the pasta to the sauté pan and toss, or place both pasta and sauce in a large serving bowl and toss.

3. To serve, chop the remaining basil leaves and sprinkle over the top.

Yields: 4 servings
Serving size: 2 cups pasta and
1 cup sauce
Calories per serving: 401

Grams of protein per serving: 14
Grams of fat per serving: 2
Milligrams of sodium per serving: 653

Recipe courtesy of Chris Bianco of Bianco's.

Pasta with Lentils and Peas

A great combination of flavors and textures gives this dish its appeal.

2 cups lentils, rinsed and picked over
4 cups water
1 pound orecchiette or other small pasta
1 medium onion, chopped
2 cloves garlic, minced
1 tablespoon olive oil

½ cup defatted chicken or vegetable stock (more as desired)
1 teaspoon red pepper flakes, optional
1 8-ounce package frozen peas, thawed
Salt to taste

1. Place the lentils and the 4 cups water in a large saucepan and bring to a boil. Then simmer, covered, about 20 to 25 minutes or until tender. Set aside.

2. Meanwhile, cook pasta according to package directions. Drain and keep warm.

3. In a large sauté pan, sauté the onion and garlic in the olive oil over medium-high heat. When lightly brown, in about 10 minutes, add the lentils, stock, and pepper flakes. Cook about 5 to 7 minutes over medium heat, stirring occasionally. Add peas and cooked pasta. Toss together in the pan or in a large serving bowl. Serve immediately.

Yields: 10 servings
Serving size: about 2 cups
Calories per serving: 292

Grams of protein per serving: 15
Grams of fat per serving: 2
Milligrams of sodium per serving: 78

Recipe courtesy of Chris Bianco of Bianco's.

Marinara Sauce

This sauce can be frozen in individual portions and reheated in the microwave for quick pasta meals.

1 tablespoon olive oil
2/3 cup minced onion
3 cloves garlic, minced
1 28-ounce can imported
   Italian tomatoes
1/2 cup unsalted tomato puree
1/4 cup chopped fresh parsley

2 teaspoons lemon zest
1/4 teaspoon freshly ground
   black pepper
1 teaspoon crushed dried
   oregano
1/2 teaspoon sugar
   Salt to taste

Heat the olive oil in a large skillet and sauté the onion and garlic in the oil over medium-high heat until soft and transparent, about 7 minutes. Add the remaining ingredients and simmer over very low heat, covered, 30 to 40 minutes, stirring frequently. During the last 10 minutes of cooking, uncover to allow sauce to thicken.

Yields: 6 servings
Serving size: 1/2 cup
Calories per serving: 77

Grams of protein per serving: 2
Grams of fat per serving: 3
Milligrams of sodium per serving: 293

Recipe courtesy of Southwest Health Institute.

Thai Noodles

Pasta with an Oriental flair!

1 12-ounce package wide rice
   noodles*
2 tablespoons vegetable oil
2 chicken breasts, skinned
   and thinly sliced
3 cloves garlic, minced
1/4 cup rice vinegar* or any
   mild vinegar
1 teaspoon fish sauce* or
   reduced-sodium soy sauce
1 tablespoon sugar
2 teaspoons ketchup

1/4 teaspoon red pepper flakes
   or 1/2 teaspoon chili
   powder
1/4 teaspoon freshly ground
   black pepper
1 egg
1/2 cup lengthwise sliced green
   onions, bulbs and greens
1 cup bean sprouts
2 tablespoons ground
   peanuts
1 lime, sliced

*These products are available in Oriental markets or the ethnic section of your supermarket.

1. Soak the noodles in warm water to cover until they are soft, about ½ hour. Drain.

2. Heat 1 tablespoon of the oil in a wok or large skillet. Add the sliced chicken and garlic. Sauté over high heat until the chicken turns white. Add the vinegar, fish sauce, sugar, ketchup, and spices and heat through over high heat.

3. Turn down the heat and stir in the softened noodles.

4. Push the ingredients to the sides, add the remaining tablespoon of oil, and stir in the egg. Cook the egg gently and then stir into the noodles.

5. Add the green onions and bean sprouts. Cook slightly over low heat, about 2 minutes. The onion and bean sprouts should remain crisp.

6. Remove to a serving platter and sprinkle with the ground peanuts. Decorate with sliced lime.

Yields: about 9 cups
Serving size: about 1½ cups
Calories per serving: 363
Grams of protein per serving: 27

Grams of fat per serving: 9 (2.5 if peanuts omitted)
Milligrams of sodium per serving: 230

Wild Risotto

RICE:

2 cups water
½ cup wild rice
½ cup brown rice

2 bay leaves
Salt and freshly ground pepper to taste

VEGETABLE MIX:

1 tablespoon olive oil
1 clove garlic, minced, optional
1 medium onion, diced
4 small carrots, diced
¼ cup apple cider

2 medium green bell peppers,
diced
¾ cup defatted chicken or
vegetable stock
2 ounces grated Parmesan
Chopped fresh parsley

1. *For rice:* In a medium saucepan, bring the water to a boil and add the rices and bay leaves. Cover and lower heat. Cook until done, about 45 minutes. Keep the rice covered throughout cooking. The rice may be done ahead 'and refrigerated.

2. *For vegetable mix:* In a large sauté pan, heat the oil and sauté the garlic, onion, and carrots over medium-high heat until light brown, about 10 minutes. Add the cider and simmer over medium heat until the liquid is reduced by half, about 15 minutes. Then add the bell peppers and the stock. Continue simmering over medium heat until the liquid is again reduced by half, about 20 minutes.

3. Remove the bay leaves from the rice. Stir the rice into the vegetable mixture and heat through.

4. Stir the Parmesan into the mixture. Garnish with chopped parsley and serve immediately.

Yields: 4 servings
Serving size: about 1½ cups
Calories per serving: 313

Grams of protein per serving: 13
Grams of fat per serving: 9
Milligrams of sodium per serving: 435

Recipe courtesy of Chris Bianco of Bianco's.

Very Important Potato (V.I.P.)

If you've had a high-protein lunch, here is an idea for a quick low-protein dinner—from microwave to plate in about 6 minutes! Serve with a green salad for a complete, tasty meal.

The topping for this keeps well for at least a week in the refrigerator, depending on the freshness of the cottage cheese when purchased.

4 potatoes (about 7 ounces each)

TOPPING:

1 cup low-fat (1%) cottage cheese

1 teaspoon chopped fresh cilantro

1 tablespoon chopped fresh chives or green onion

1/8 teaspoon dried dill

Dash of Tabasco or other hot pepper sauce, optional

1/8 teaspoon paprika

Salt if desired (remember that cottage cheese is relatively high in sodium)

1. Scrub potatoes well. Bake in a 350°F oven for 1 hour until done or microwave potatoes for 7 minutes each until done.

2. For topping: Whip the cottage cheese in a blender until smooth. Add the herbs and spices and blend briefly until mixed.

3. Cut a cross in each baked potato and top each with 1/4 cup of cheese topping. Sprinkle with paprika.

Yields: 4 servings
Serving size: 1 potato and 1/4 cup cheese topping
Calories per serving: 262

Grams of protein per serving: 12
Grams of fat per serving: 1
Milligrams of sodium per serving: 246

Recipe courtesy of Southwest Health Institute.

Chapter 16

Innovative Vegetables

Almond Broccoli

1¼ pounds fresh broccoli
2 cloves garlic, minced
1 tablespoon olive oil

2 tablespoons chopped almonds
Juice of 1 lemon
⅓ cup sliced pitted black olives

1. Break the broccoli into stems and steam until just tender, about 5 minutes. Remove to a serving platter.

2. In a skillet, sauté the garlic in the olive oil over medium-high heat until soft, about 2 minutes. Add the almonds, the lemon juice, and sliced olives. Heat through.

3. Pour the garlic mixture over the broccoli and serve warm.

Yields: about 4 cups
Serving size: ⅔ cup
Calories per serving: 60
Grams of protein per serving: 3

Grams of fat per serving: 4 (2 if almonds are omitted)
Milligrams of sodium per serving: 33

Recipe courtesy of Southwest Health Institute.

Marinated Carrots

This marinade can be reserved and used again on another of your favorite vegetables.

7 large carrots, cut into thick julienne strips
¼ cup olive oil
¼ cup rice vinegar* or any mild vinegar
½ cup thin strips green onions, bulbs and tops
2 whole cloves garlic
2 tablespoons pimentos

2 teaspoons minced fresh basil
2 tablespoons fresh lemon or lime juice
¼ cup water
¼ teaspoon freshly ground black pepper
1 teaspoon salt, optional
Salad greens

1. Steam or microwave the carrot strips until just barely tender, about 4 minutes.

2. Combine the remaining ingredients in a large glass bowl. Add the carrots and marinate, covered, for approximately 12 hours.

3. Drain and reserve the marinade, remove the garlic, serve the carrots on a bed of salad greens, and sprinkle with some of the marinade if you wish.

Yields: 8 servings
Serving size: ½ cup
Calories per serving: 95
Grams of protein per serving: 1

Grams of fat per serving: 2
Milligrams of sodium per serving: 165 (23 if salt is not added)

Recipe courtesy of Southwest Health Institute.
*Rice vinegar is available in Oriental markets or the ethnic section of your supermarket.

Squash and Apple Bake

Even those who think they don't like squash will want a second helping of this dish.

Nonstick vegetable spray
1 2-pound butternut squash, peeled, seeded, and cut into slices
4 medium-size tart apples

(Granny Smith), peeled and sliced
1 teaspoon cinnamon
2 tablespoons brown sugar
2 teaspoons vegetable oil

1. Spray an 8-inch square glass baking dish with nonstick spray.
2. Arrange the squash slices evenly in the baking dish. Top with apple slices. Sprinkle the cinnamon and brown sugar evenly over the apples. Drizzle the vegetable oil evenly over all.
3. Cover and bake in a 350° oven for 30 minutes or in a microwave on high for 10 minutes. Turn the dish one-quarter turn and microwave an additional 5 minutes or until the squash is tender.

Yields: about 6 cups
Serving size: 1 cup
Calories per serving: 124

Grams of protein per serving: 2
Grams of fat per serving: 2
Milligrams of sodium per serving: 25

Recipe courtesy of Southwest Health Institute.

Spaghetti Squash with Tomato, Basil, and Garlic Sauce

Here is another way to get a great meal from the Tomato, Basil, and Garlic Sauce on page 245.

1 spaghetti squash (about 5 pounds)

1 recipe Tomato, Basil, and Garlic Sauce (page 245)
Chopped fresh basil

1. Preheat oven to 350°F.
2. With a fork, punch a few holes in the squash. Place it in the oven on a cookie sheet for 45 to 50 minutes. Remove from the

oven and carefully cut in half lengthwise. Remove the seeds. With a fork, scrape out the flesh of the squash—it will resemble strands of spaghetti—into a large bowl.

3. Add just enough of the Tomato, Basil, and Garlic Sauce to coat the squash, and toss.

4. To serve, top with chopped fresh basil.

Yields: 4 servings
Serving size: about 2 cups squash and 1 cup sauce
Calories per serving: 277

Grams of protein per serving: 8
Grams of fat per serving: 4
Milligrams of sodium per serving: 747

Recipe courtesy of Chris Bianco of Bianco's.

Fiery Tomatoes

Serve these on a bed of thinly sliced mixed lettuces or on whole endive leaves—very pretty!

1½ **pounds ripe tomatoes (about 3 large)**
½ **green bell pepper**
1 **medium red onion**
¼ **cup sliced celery**
⅓ **cup rice vinegar* or any mild vinegar**

⅛ **teaspoon freshly ground black pepper**
Dash of Tabasco or other hot pepper sauce
¾ **teaspoon mustard seed**
2 **teaspoons sugar**
¼ **cup ice water**

1. Dip the tomatoes briefly into boiling water. Peel them and cut them into bite-size wedges. Slice the onion into rings. Arrange the vegetables in a shallow glass dish.

2. In another bowl, mix together the vinegar, spices, sugar, and water and pour over the vegetables. Allow to marinate, covered in the refrigerator, for several hours.

Yields: 4 servings
Serving size: about 1 cup
Calories per serving: 61

Grams of protein per serving: 2
Grams of fat per serving: 1
Milligrams of sodium per serving: 23

Recipe courtesy of Southwest Health Institute.
*Rice vinegar is available at Oriental markets or the ethnic section of your supermarket.

Chapter 17

Protein Once a Day

Fish, chicken, and beef are all comparable in protein content, but they do have different amounts and types of fat. Saturated fat (the type that raises your blood cholesterol) should be eaten in small quantities—less than 10 percent of your total fat allowance for the day should be saturated fat.

Egg yolks contain a considerable amount of cholesterol. When you are using eggs in cooking, you may substitute two egg whites for every egg yolk.

Because the Anti-Aging Diet intends to provide you with a workable eating pattern for the rest of your life, we feature sensible recipes that use animal protein as their main ingredient. Integrating a beef recipe into your meal plan once a week and fish, chicken, or egg two to four times a week—depending on your goal weight—should provide enough variety to keep you interested as well as healthy.

Remember: Protein should be a side dish, not a main dish. These great recipes will show you the way to begin changing even the most confirmed meat eater's tastes and habits.

Broiled Marinated Shrimp

This makes an elegant meal served on a bed of your favorite pasta and accompanied by our Almond Broccoli (page 251).

¼ cup fresh lemon juice
1 tablespoon vegetable oil
1 teaspoon Worcestershire sauce
¼ teaspoon Tabasco or other hot pepper sauce

¾ cup fine dry breadcrumbs
1 pound large fresh or frozen shrimp, shelled and deveined

1. Combine the lemon juice, oil, and sauces in a shallow glass dish. Marinate the shrimp in this mixture, covered in the refrigerator, about 4 hours.
2. Preheat the broiler for a few minutes.
3. Drain the shrimp and roll in the breadcrumbs. Broil about 3 minutes on one side, turn, and broil about 3 minutes on the other side. Do not overcook. Shrimp will turn pink when done.

Yields: 4 servings
Serving size: 4 ounces shrimp
Calories per serving: 216

Grams of protein per serving: 23
Grams of fat per serving: 5
Milligrams of sodium per serving: 309

Recipe courtesy of Southwest Health Institute.

Herbed Red Snapper

1 pound Pacific red snapper or other firm fish fillets
1 teaspoon dried marjoram
1 teaspoon onion powder
½ teaspoon paprika

¼ teaspoon coarsely ground black pepper
1 tablespoon fresh parsley
1 teaspoon olive oil
2 tablespoons fresh lime juice

1. Preheat oven to 375°F.
2. Remove any bones from the fish, wash, and pat dry with paper towels. Place the fish in an ovenproof dish.

3. Combine the herbs and spices in a bowl and sprinkle evenly over the fish.

4. Combine the olive oil and lime juice in a bowl. Drizzle over the fish.

5. Cover and bake about 20 minutes or until the fish flakes with a fork.

Yields: 4 servings

Serving size: 4 ounces snapper

Calories per serving: 164

Grams of protein per serving: 27

Grams of fat per serving: 6

Milligrams of sodium per serving: 127

Recipe courtesy of Southwest Health Institute.

Fish Naranja

This elegant dish can also be made with chicken instead of fish, but be sure to add an extra 15 minutes to the cooking time to insure that the chicken is sufficiently cooked.

2 teaspoons orange zest

2 cups orange juice

¼ cup reduced-sodium soy sauce

2 teaspoons minced fresh ginger

4 carrots, julienne sliced

1½ pounds white fish fillets (cod, orange roughy, or haddock)

2 cups unpeeled, julienne-cut zucchini

½ cup apple cider

1. Combine the orange zest, orange juice, soy sauce, and ginger in a large skillet. Cook over medium heat for 1 minute. Add the carrots and continue cooking over medium heat for 5 minutes. Reduce the heat to a simmer, push the carrots to the outer edge of the skillet, and add the fish. Arrange the zucchini around the fish. Cover and simmer about 5 minutes, or until the fish flakes easily with a fork.

2. Remove the fish and vegetables to a platter, using a slotted

spoon, and keep warm. Add the apple cider to the liquid in the skillet, stir, and gently simmer for a few minutes.

3. To serve, spoon the liquid over the fish and vegetables.

Yields: 8 servings
Serving size: 3 ounces fish and ½ cup vegetables
Calories per serving: 126

Grams of protein per serving: 17
Grams of fat per serving: 1
Milligrams of sodium per serving: 321

Recipe courtesy of Southwest Health Institute.

Apple Salmon and Sauerkraut en Papillotte

Sweet and sour blend beautifully to enhance the flavor of the fish.

4   5-ounce salmon fillets or steaks
2   tablespoons Dijon mustard
    Juice of 1 lemon
¼   cup fresh apple cider
4   cloves garlic, chopped

1   12-ounce can low-sodium sauerkraut, drained
2   tablespoons chopped fresh dill
1   Red Delicious apple, cored and sliced

1. Preheat oven to 500°F.
2. Remove the skin and bones from the salmon pieces and rinse them with cold water. Pat dry with paper towels. Set aside.
3. Mix together in a small bowl the mustard, lemon juice, cider, and garlic. Set aside.
4. Tear off 4 pieces of aluminum foil, each 8 to 10 inches long. Place one fourth of the sauerkraut in the center of each piece of foil. Place the salmon on top of the sauerkraut. Spoon one fourth of the cider mixture over each piece of salmon and top with the fresh dill. Arrange a few apple slices around each piece of fish. Seal the foil tightly over the fish but leave some room between the edge of the package and the salmon.
5. Place on a cookie sheet and bake 10 minutes. Serve.

Yields: 4 servings   Grams of protein per serving: 33
Serving size: 1 papillotte   Grams of fat per serving: 19
Calories per serving: 361   Milligrams of sodium per serving: 600

Recipe courtesy of Chris Bianco of Bianco's.

Foil-Baked Citrus Sea Bass

This is a foolproof method of cooking fish.

4 5-ounce sea bass or orange roughy fillets

MARINADE:

Juice of 1 orange, 1 lemon,
or 1 lime
1 tablespoon Worcester-
shire sauce
1 teaspoon paprika
4 green onions, bulbs and
tops, chopped

8 fresh basil leaves, torn
1 teaspoon dried Greek
oregano
¼ cup dry white wine
Salt and freshly ground
black pepper

1. Preheat oven to 500°F.
2. Wash the fish fillets in cold water and pat them dry with paper towels.
3. Mix together the marinade ingredients in a shallow dish or bowl, adding salt and freshly ground black pepper to taste. Add the sea bass fillets and marinate about 20 minutes.
4. Remove the fillets and place each on a piece of aluminum foil big enough to fold over and seal around the fish. Spoon some of the marinade over each fillet, making sure you arrange some of the green onions and basil on top of each portion of the fish.
5. Seal the foil around the fish, making sure there are no holes. Place the fish on a cookie sheet and bake for 10 minutes. Remove from packages to serve.

Yields: 4 servings
Serving size: 5-ounce sea bass
  fillet
Calories per serving: 173

Grams of protein per serving: 31
Grams of fat per serving: 1
Milligrams of sodium per serving: 144

Recipe courtesy of Chris Bianco of Bianco's.

Christopher's Fish Soup

(The fish should all be cut to approximately the same thickness so the cooking time will be the same.)

1 fennel bulb
3 cups dry white wine
7 cloves garlic, crushed
1 medium onion, thinly
   sliced
2 stalks celery, chopped
6 medium tomatoes, chopped
   and seeded, or 2 28-ounce
   cans unsalted tomatoes,
   drained and chopped
1 sprig fresh thyme
¼ teaspoon saffron threads
¼ cup chopped fresh parsley
2 cups water

3 pounds heads and bones of
   white-fleshed fish, such as
   sole, halibut, or turbot
8 ounces scallops
8 ounces mahi-mahi or
   swordfish, cut into bite-size
   pieces
8 ounces salmon fillet, cut
   into bite-size pieces
   Salt and freshly ground
   white pepper
6 ½-inch-thick slices of
   French bread, toasted

1. Cut off the top of the fennel bulb and remove the small tough core. Slice the bulb into the thinnest rings possible.

2. In a large soup pot, gently heat ½ cup of the wine and "sweat" 6 of the garlic cloves (set aside 1 clove), the fennel, onion, and celery until softened, about 5 minutes.

3. Add the tomatoes, thyme, saffron, parsley, water, the remaining 2½ cups of wine, and the fish heads and bones wrapped in cheese cloth bag. Bring to a boil. Reduce the heat to low and simmer for 45 minutes, skimming any foam.

4. Remove the fish heads and bones and discard them. Puree the

soup in batches in a food processor or blender. Then strain the soup through a fine sieve back into the soup pot. Boil the soup vigorously for about 20 minutes, or until slightly thickened and reduced to about 6 cups.

5. Reduce the heat to low and add the scallops, mahi-mahi, and salmon. Simmer, uncovered, for 2 to 4 minutes, or until the fish flesh is opaque. Season with salt and freshly ground white pepper to taste.

6. Toast the bread slices in a 350°F oven until they begin to color, about 10 minutes. Rub each with the remaining garlic clove.

7. To serve, place a piece of toast on the bottom of a large soup bowl and ladle 2 cups of soup over it.

Yields: 6 servings   *Grams of protein per serving: 30*
Serving size: about 2 cups   *Grams of fat per serving: 9*
Calories per serving: 324   *Milligrams of sodium per serving: 220*

Recipe courtesy of Christopher Gross of Christopher's.

Grilled Breast of Chicken with Jicama and Sweet Peppers in Sherry Wine Vinegar Sauce

6 4-ounces boneless chicken breast halves, skin and all inside fat removed

Freshly ground black pepper
Olive oil

SHERRY WINE VINEGAR SAUCE:

½ cup sherry wine vinegar
1 tablespoon defatted chicken stock

4 tablespoons olive oil
Salt and freshly ground black pepper

JICAMA AND PEPPERS:

1 tablespoon olive oil
1 small jicama,* peeled and
shredded
1 red bell pepper, chopped

1 yellow bell pepper,
chopped
1 green bell pepper, chopped

1. Season the chicken breasts with pepper and lightly brush them with olive oil. Grill for 8 minutes on each side. Remove the breasts and keep warm.

2. *For sherry wine vinegar sauce:* Boil the vinegar in a small saucepan over high heat until it has reduced by half, about 10 minutes. Stir in the chicken stock and 4 tablespoons of olive oil. Add salt and freshly ground black pepper to taste and keep warm over low heat until ready to serve.

3. In a sauté pan, heat the tablespoon of olive oil and sauté the shredded jicama for approximately 2 minutes; remove. In the same pan, sauté the bell peppers for approximately 2 minutes.

4. To serve, evenly divide the jicama into 6 portions and place on serving plates. Top each serving with a chicken breast. Arrange the bell peppers equally and evenly around the sides. Serve hot with sherry wine vinegar sauce on the side.

Yields: 6 servings
Serving size: 4-ounce chicken breast
Calories per serving: 343

Grams of protein per serving: 25
Grams of fat per serving: 18 (to decrease the fat per serving, go easy on the sauce)
Milligrams of sodium per serving: 85

Recipe courtesy of Vincent Guerithault of Vincent's on Camelback.
*Jicama is available in Spanish bodegas or supermarkets. Use potato, turnip, or water chestnuts if jicama is not available.

Chicken Fajitas

Serve these with Fresh Salsa (page 223) or Salsa Pronto (page 224) and Spanish rice.

1 tablespoon olive oil
3 12-ounce boneless chicken breasts, skin and all visible fat removed; cut into strips
1 medium zucchini, cut into thin strips
1 green bell pepper, cut into strips

1 medium onion, sliced
2 cloves garlic, minced
½ teaspoon fresh cilantro or pinch of dried cilantro
2 teaspoons chili powder
Pinch of red pepper flakes, optional
6 6-inch flour tortillas

1. Heat the oil in a skillet and stir fry the chicken strips in the oil over medium-high heat until the chicken turns white, about 5 minutes.

2. Add the remaining ingredients, except the tortillas, and stir fry over medium-high heat until the vegetables are crisp tender, about 5 minutes.

3. Divide the mixture evenly into 6 servings. Place a serving of the chicken mixture in the center of each tortilla. Fold the tortilla over in half to form the fajita.

Yields: 6 servings
Serving size: 1 fajita, 6 ounces chicken
Calories per serving: 169

Grams of protein per serving: 18
Grams of fat per serving: 5
Milligrams of sodium per serving: 69

Recipe courtesy of Southwest Health Institute.

Chicken Chalupas

This is a fun meal in which each person creates his own colorful chalupa from an assortment of fresh toppings. And, of course, pass the Fresh Salsa (page 223) or Salsa Pronto (page 224). Fresh fruit completes this meal.

1 pound dried pinto beans, rinsed and picked over

12 cups water

1 pound boneless chicken breasts, skin and all visible fat removed

4 cloves garlic, chopped

2 4-ounce cans mild green chilies, chopped

2 tablespoons chili powder

1 tablespoon ground cumin

1 teaspoon dried oregano

GARNISH:

12 6-inch corn tortillas
Tomatoes, chopped
Green onions, bulbs and tops, chopped
Onions, chopped

Lettuce, shredded
Green bell peppers, chopped
Jalapeño peppers, sliced

1. Put the beans into a large soup pot with 12 cups of water, cover, and allow to soak overnight.

2. The next day, do not drain. Add all the other ingredients except the garnishes, cover, and simmer over very low heat until the beans are soft, about 4 hours, stirring occasionally. During the last hour of cooking, remove the lid so the mixture can thicken. Continue to stir occasionally.

3. Place tortillas in a preheated oven at 350° for 3 minutes to crisp.

4. Pile each tortilla with the mixture and provide an assortment of garnishes. Or put a tortilla and 1 cup of the bean mixture on each plate and pass the garnishes.

Yields: 12 servings
Serving size: 1 cup + 1 cup garnish + 1 tortilla
Calories per serving: 273

Grams of protein per serving: 24
Grams of fat per serving: 2
Milligrams of sodium per serving: 120

Recipe courtesy of Chris Bianco of Bianco's.

Lemon Garlic Chicken Paillards

Serve these with a large green salad and country-style bread.

4 5-ounce boneless chicken breast halves, skin and all visible fat removed

MARINADE:

4 cloves garlic, minced
1 tablespoon chopped
fresh cilantro
1/4 teaspoon red pepper flakes,
optional

1 teaspoon fresh oregano
Salt
Juice of 1 lemon or 1
orange or 2 limes
1/4 cup olive oil

1. One at a time, place each chicken breast between two pieces of waxed paper or parchment. Pound the chicken with a meat tenderizer or mallet until the desired thinness is achieved (breast should almost double in size). Repeat with each chicken breast.

2. *For marinade:* In a shallow dish or bowl mix together the garlic, cilantro, red pepper flakes, salt to taste, oregano, fruit juice, and olive oil.

3. Place the prepared breasts in the marinade and allow to marinate in the refrigerator for 2 hours, turning once.

4. Prepare charcoal or gas grill. Remove the chicken from the marinade and grill about 4 minutes on each side. Because they are thin, they will cook very fast.

5. Serve immediately.

Yields: 4 servings
Serving size: 1 5-ounce
chicken breast
Calories per serving: 372

Grams of protein per serving: 40
Grams of fat per serving: 10
Milligrams of sodium per serving: 111

Recipe courtesy of Chris Bianco of Bianco's.

Grilled Chicken Breasts with Couscous Salad

The couscous salad is pungent and peppery. For variety, try it with grilled fish or canned tuna.

2 boneless chicken breasts,
   skin and all visible fat removed

1 teaspoon olive oil

HARISSA (RED PEPPER SAUCE):

3 red bell peppers
2 cloves garlic
1 tablespoon chopped onion

3 drops chili oil or to taste
   Pinch of cayenne pepper

COUSCOUS:

1 cup couscous
1½ cups boiling water
2 tablespoons plus
2 teapoons olive oil
½ cup sliced fresh shiitake or
   domestic mushrooms
2½ tablespoons defatted
   chicken or vegetable stock
2 tablespoons balsamic vinegar

⅛ teaspoon salt, optional
¼ cup chopped arugula or
   watercress leaves
1 medium tomato, peeled,
   seeded, and diced
2 tablespoons minced chives
2 tablespoons pine nuts
   Fresh parsley sprigs for
   garnish

1. Brush 1 teaspoon olive oil on the chicken and grill about 3 minutes on each side or until cooked. When cooked, remove from the grill and refrigerate. These can be cooked ahead and stored in the refrigerator for up to 2 days.

2. *For harissa:* Place the peppers under the broiler, about 4 inches from heat, for about 10 minutes or until they are blackened all over. Place them in a paper bag and set aside for about 15 minutes. Peel off and discard the skin and discard the membrane and seeds. Chop the flesh coarsely and place in a food processor or blender along with the garlic, onion, chili oil, and cayenne. Process until smooth. The sauce can be made ahead and stored in the refrigerator for up to 2 days.

3. Place the couscous in a shallow heatproof dish. Stir in the

boiling water and 1 teaspoon olive oil. Cover and let stand for 10 minutes. Fluff with a fork, then refrigerate until cool.

4. In a small nonstick skillet, heat 1 teaspoon olive oil. Add the mushrooms and sauté for 2 to 3 minutes, or until softened. Set aside to cool.

5. In a small bowl, whisk together the chicken stock, vinegar, and ⅛ teaspoon salt if desired. Gradually whisk in the 2 tablespoons olive oil. Set aside.

6. In a large bowl, gently toss together ½ cup of the harissa, the couscous, mushrooms, arugula, tomato, and chives. Toss the pine nuts in a skillet over high heat for 2 minutes to toast and add to the couscous mixture.

7. To serve, mold 1 cup of the couscous in a 4-inch-diameter mound on a serving plate. Slice the chicken thinly, divide into 4 servings, and arrange each portion in a fan pattern over the couscous. Garnish with parsley and serve with additional harissa.

Yields: 4 servings
Serving size: 2 ounces
chicken and about 1 cup
salad

Calories per serving: 423
Grams of protein per serving: 24
Grams of fat per serving: 16
Milligrams of sodium per serving: 78

Recipe courtesy of Christopher Gross of Christopher's.

Lentil and Wheat Berry Ossobucco

2 tablespoons olive oil
6 veal shanks*, each about 2 inches thick (about 24 ounces total)
Freshly ground black pepper
1 medium carrot, diced
1 medium onion, diced
2 stalks celery, diced
5 cloves garlic, minced
1¼ cups dry white wine
1 sprig fresh thyme, snipped

1 bay leaf
1 sprig fresh parsley, snipped
6 leaves fresh basil, chopped
4 medium tomatoes, halved and seeded
1 to 2 cups defatted chicken stock or water
½ cup wheat berries
½ cup tiny green lentils, rinsed and picked over
Salt

1. Preheat oven to 350°F.

2. Heat 1 tablespoon olive oil in a skillet. Season the veal with freshly ground black pepper, if desired, and brown in the oil over medium-high heat. When browned, transfer the veal to an oven-proof casserole dish.

3. Heat the rest of the olive oil in the skillet and sauté the carrot, onion, celery, and garlic over medium-high heat about 2 minutes. Transfer the vegetables to the casserole dish.

4. Use the wine to deglaze the sauté pan. Then pour the wine over the veal and vegetables. Add the thyme, bay leaf, parsley, basil, and tomatoes to the casserole. Add enough chicken stock or water to cover the veal. Cover the casserole and bake until the veal is very tender, about 1½ hours.

5. Meanwhile, cover the wheat berries with water in a small saucepan and simmer until tender, about 1 hour. Cover the lentils with water in a small saucepan and cook over low heat until tender, about 30 minutes.

6. When the veal is done, remove it to a platter and keep hot. Strain the sauce into a saucepan. Reduce the sauce by simmering until it has reached a nice consistency. Add the cooked wheat berries and lentils. Season with salt and pepper if desired.

7. To serve, top the hot veal with sauce, wheat berries, and lentils.

Yields: 6 servings　　　　　*Grams of protein per serving: 29*
Serving size: 4 ounces veal　*Grams of fat per serving: 11*
Calories per serving: 339　　*Milligrams of sodium per serving: 110*

Recipe courtesy of Christopher Gross of Christopher's.

*Christopher recommends purchasing the veal from Summerfield Farm, which offers mail-order service. Call (703) 948-3100 or write Summerfield Farm, HCR 4, Box 195A, Brightwood, VA 22715.

Huevos Rancheros (Ranch-Style Eggs)

Surround this brunch item with a colorful array of fresh fruits.

1 cup cooked pinto beans or canned vegetarian-style refried beans

2 tablespoons nonfat plain yogurt

4 6-inch corn tortillas

4 whole eggs

½ tablespoon vegetable oil

1 cup Fresh Salsa (page 223) or Salsa Pronto (page 224)

4 tablespoons shredded low-fat Monterey Jack cheese

Shredded lettuce

1. Preheat oven to 350°F.

2. Process cooked pinto beans in a food processor until a semi-smooth paste is formed. If using the canned refried beans, omit this step.

3. Mix the beans and the yogurt together in a small bowl and set aside.

4. Place the tortillas on a cookie sheet and brush a small amount of the vegetable oil on each tortilla. (If you use prepackaged hard corn tortillas, omit the oil.) Heat the tortillas in the oven until sizzling, about 8 minutes.

5. Spread one quarter of the bean mixture on each tortilla and return to the oven to heat the beans, about 5 minutes.

6. Meanwhile, brush a small amount of the oil on a nonstick skillet or griddle and cook the eggs. Turn the eggs over to cook the white completely. The yolk should be thoroughly heated but still partially liquid.

7. Top each tortilla with one cooked egg. Top each egg with one quarter of the salsa and sprinkle with 1 tablespoon of cheese. Return to the warm oven until the cheese is slightly melted.

8. Serve on a bed of shredded lettuce.

Yields: 4 servings

Serving size: 1 egg

Calories per serving: 241

Grams of protein per serving: 15

Grams of fat per serving: 11

Milligrams of sodium per serving: 200

Recipe courtesy of Southwest Health Institute.

Chapter 18

Sweets

Zabaglione

⅓ cup evaporated skim milk,
   well chilled
2 tablespoons confectioners'
   sugar
2 tablespoons vanilla nonfat
   yogurt
1 tablespoon Marsala

1 tablespoon sherry
2 tablespoons grated orange
   rind or lemon zest
1 teaspoon vanilla extract
1 quart berries, mixed or one
   of your choice

1. Whip the chilled evaporated milk until creamy.

2. In a bowl, mix together the yogurt, Marsala, rind or zest, and vanilla together. Fold into the whipped milk.

3. Divide the berries equally into 4 individual heatproof serving bowls. Spoon equal amounts of the yogurt mixture over the berries in each bowl and then brown under the broiler for a few seconds or until golden and crispy brown. Serve immediately.

Yields: *4 servings*
Serving size: *about ¾ cup*
Calories per serving: *97*

Grams of protein per serving: *3*
Grams of fat per serving: *1*
Milligrams of sodium per serving: *31*

Recipe courtesy of Benito of Avanti's.

Mollen Shake

1 banana
1 cup fresh or frozen whole strawberries
1 cup plain nonfat yogurt
1 cup crushed ice

1 cup skim milk or more if desired
1 teaspoon strawberry preserves

Combine all the ingredients in a blender and blend until smooth. If the shake is too thick, add a small amount of skim milk until it is the consistency you desire.

Yields: *about 1 quart*
Serving size: *about 10 ounces*
Calories per serving: *132*

Grams of protein per serving: *8*
Grams of fat per serving: *0.5*
Milligrams of sodium per serving: *106*

Recipe courtesy of Southwest Health Institute.

Ricottacakes

These are wonderful with sliced strawberries, whole blueberries, or sliced apples. If allowed, you may use a little syrup.

1 pound part-skim ricotta
1⅓ cups skim milk
2 teaspoons baking powder*
1 cup whole wheat flour

6 egg whites, at room temperature
Vegetable oil or nonstick vegetable spray
Cinnamon

1. Blend the ricotta and milk on high speed in a blender until smooth. Reduce the speed and mix in the baking powder and flour. Blend until smooth.

2. In a separate bowl, whip the egg whites until stiff, but not dry. Transfer the ricotta mixture to a large bowl and gently fold in the egg whites.

3. Lightly oil or spray a pancake griddle or frying pan. Heat the griddle and bake the pancakes on the hot griddle, using ¼ cup of batter per pancake. Turn the pancake when golden brown and continue cooking until golden brown on the other side.

4. Serve with a sprinkling of cinnamon.

Yields: 8 servings   *Grams of protein per serving: 12*
Serving size: 3 pancakes   *Grams of fat per serving: 5*
Calories per serving: 155   *Milligrams of sodium per serving: 235*

Recipe courtesy of Southwest Health Institute.
*To eliminate the bitter taste, use a calcium-based baking powder rather than an aluminum-based one.

Native American Roast Pineapple

This dessert is delicious eaten as is, or it can be served over frozen yogurt or sherbet.

1 large fresh pineapple   2 teaspoons cinnamon
¼ cup orange juice
2 tablespoons orange blos-
    som or other honey

1. Preheat oven to 425°F.

2. Cut the pineapple in half lengthwise and remove the core. There will be a U-shaped indentation down the center of the pineapple. Score the fruit deeply into squares, cutting the flesh loose.

3. Mix the orange juice and honey together in a bowl and spoon over the fruit. Top with the cinnamon.

4. Place the pineapple halves, fruit side up, on a cookie sheet and bake in the oven for 20 minutes.

5. To serve, remove the fruit and place about ¾ cup in each serving dish with the juices spooned over.

Yields: 6 to 8 servings	*Grams of protein per serving: 0*
Serving size: about ¾ cup	*Grams of fat per serving: 0*
Calories per serving: 78	*Milligrams of sodium per serving: 2*

Recipe courtesy of Chris Bianco of Bianco's.

Pastel Requeso'n (Kiwi-Crowned Cottage Cheese Pie)

This attractive dessert is high in protein and should only follow a low-protein meal.

1½ cups Grape Nuts cereal	½ cup skim milk
1 tablespoon vegetable oil	1 teaspoon vanilla extract
2 cups nonfat cottage cheese	2 teaspoons lemon zest
2 egg whites	4 kiwi, sliced
⅓ cup sugar	

1. Preheat oven to 350°F.

2. Blend the Grape Nuts cereal and the oil together in a bowl. Pat the mixture into the bottom of a 9-inch-square glass baking dish. Bake about 6 minutes or until browned. Cool.

3. In an electric blender or food processor, mix the remaining ingredients except kiwi until the cottage cheese is smooth.

4. Pour the pie filling over the cooled crust and return to the oven for about 20 minutes, or until set.

5. To serve, cut into squares and decorate the top of each serving with an equal amount of sliced kiwi.

Yields: 9 servings	*Grams of protein per serving: 10*
Serving size: 1 3-inch square	*Grams of fat per serving: 5*
Calories per serving: 204	*Milligrams of sodium per serving: 394*

Recipe courtesy of Southwest Health Institute.

Fromage Blanc with Coconut Pastry and Puree of Strawberries

COCONUT PASTRY:

1 cup sugar
¾ cup all-purpose flour
3 tablespoons canola oil
½ teaspoon vanilla extract or more to taste
1 generous pint fresh strawberries

14 to 16 ounces fromage blanc* or part-skim ricotta
8 fluid ounces egg whites (4 or 5 eggs)
2 tablespoons unsweetened shredded coconut

1. Preheat oven to 350°F.

2. *For coconut pastry:* In a large bowl, mix together until well blended the sugar, flour, oil, and vanilla. Then add the egg whites and mix until smooth.

3. Spread a very thin coat of the paste on a Teflon-coated, ovenproof pan or cookie sheet and sprinkle with the coconut. Bake in the oven until the paste becomes light brown, about 3 to 5 minutes. Remove the pan from the oven and flip the pan over onto a clean cutting surface, allowing the paste sheet to fall out of the pan. Immediately cut it into 2½-inch-wide strips and roll these strips quickly into tube shapes around a wooden dowel about 1½ inches in diameter. Trim off any excess pastry. Let cool.

4. Clean, hull, puree, and strain the strawberries. Refrigerate the puree.

5. Using a pastry bag without a tip, fill the pastry tubes with fromage blanc. To serve, garnish each tube with one eighth of the strawberry puree.

Yields: 8 pastries
Serving size: 1 pastry
Calories per serving: 293

Grams of protein per serving: 12
Grams of fat per serving: 11
Milligrams of sodium per serving: 131

Recipe courtesy of Christopher Gross of Christopher's.
*Fromage blanc is a soft white cheese available at gourmet shops.

Peach Sorbet

2 **pounds fresh, ripe peaches**
4 **tablespoons fresh lemon
   juice**

⅓ **cup orange blossom or
   other honey**
1 **cup water**

1. Bring a large pot of water to a boil. Blanch the peaches in the boiling water for 25 seconds, then immediately place in an ice bath. Skin and pit the peaches.

2. In a blender or food processor, blend the peaches and the lemon juice for about 1 minute. Refrigerate.

3. In a large saucepan, combine the honey and water. Bring to a boil—the mixture will "bubble up" to about twice its original volume. Reduce the heat and let simmer about 10 minutes, stirring occasionally. Remove from the heat and let cool.

4. Blend together the peach puree and the honey mixture. Transfer to an ice cream maker and follow manufacturer's directions.

Yields: 6 servings
Serving size: about 1 cup
Calories per serving: 124

Grams of protein per serving: 1
Grams of fat per serving: 0
Milligrams of sodium per serving: 1

Recipe courtesy of Chris Bianco of Bianco's.

NOTES

Chapter 2: The Search for a Revolutionary Diet

1. Robert C. Atkins, *Dr. Atkins' Diet Revolution* (New York: Bantam Books, 1973).

2. Russell H. Chittenden, *Physiological Economy in Nutrition* (New York: Frederick A. Stokes, 1904).

3. Clive M. McCay et al., "The Life Span of Rats on a Restricted Diet," *Journal of Nutrition* 18 (1939):1–25.

4. Clive M. McCay, "Effect of Restricted Feeding upon Aging and Chronic Diseases in Rats and Dogs," *American Journal of Public Health* 37 (1947):521.

5. J. Bergstrom and E. Hultman, "Muscle Glycogen Synthesis in Relation to Diet Studied in Normal Subjects," *Acta Medica Scandinavica* 182 (1967): 107–117; B. Ahlborg et al., "Muscle Glycogen and Muscle Electrolytes During Prolonged Physical Exercise," *Acta Physiologica Scandinavica* 70 (1967): 129–142.

6. Richard B. Mazess and Warren Mather, "Bone Mineral Content of North Alaskan Eskimos," *American Journal of Clinical Nutrition* 27 (1974): 916–925.

7. Clyde Williams, "Diet and Endurance Fitness," *American Journal of Clinical Nutrition* 49 (1989): 1077–1083.

8. Ronda C. Bell et al., "NK Cell Activity and Dietary Protein Intake in an Aflatoxin B1 [AF]-Induced Tumor Model," *FASEB Journal (Federation of American Societies for Experimental Biology)* Abstract No. 4511, 1990.

Chapter 3: The Overrated Protein

1. Arthur C. Guyton, *Physiology of the Body* (Philadelphia: W. B. Saunders, 1964).

2. M. Isabel Irwin and D. Mark Hegsted, "A Conspectus of Research on Protein Requirements of Man," *The Journal of Nutrition* 101 (1971): 385–430.

3. Vernon R. Young and Peter L. Pellett, "Protein Intake and Requirements with Reference to Diet and Health," *American Journal of Clinical Nutrition* 45 (1987): 1323–1343.

4. Barry M. Brenner et al., "Dietary Protein Intake and the Progressive Nature of Kidney Disease," *New England Journal of Medicine* 307 (1982): 652–659.

5. Roy Walford, "The Clinical Promise of Diet Restriction," *Geriatrics* 45 (1990): 81–83, 86–87.

6. Brenner et al., *op. cit.*

7. T. Addis, *Glomerular Nephritis: Diagnosis and Treatment* (New York: Macmillan, 1948).

8. Benno U. Ihle et al., "The Effect of Protein Restriction on the Progression of Renal Insufficiency," *New England Journal of Medicine* 321 (1989): 1773–1777.

9. John W. Kusek et al., Modification of Diet in Renal Disease (MDRD) Study Group. "An Overview of the Modification of Diet in Renal Disease Study." Nutritional and Pharmacological Strategies in Chronic Renal Failure. *Contributions in Nephrology* 81 (1990): 50–60.

10. Mazess and Mather, "Bone Content of Eskimos."

11. F. R. Ellis et al., "Incidence of Osteoporosis in Vegetarians and Omnivores," *American Journal of Clinical Nutrition* 6 (1972): 555–558.

12. M. Iguchi et al., "Clinical Effects of Prophylactic Dietary Treatment on Renal Stones," *Journal of Urology* 144 (1990): 229–232; Wanda A. Firth and Richard W. Norman, "The Effects of Modified Diets on Urinary Risk Factors for Kidney Stone Disease," *Journal of the Canadian Dietetic Association* 51 (1990): 404–408.

13. R. O. Sinnhuber, "Low-Protein Diets and Carcienogenesis of the Liver in the Trout," *Journal of the National Cancer Institute* 60 (1977): 317–320.

14. B. Scott Appleton and T. Colin Campbell, "Inhibition of Aflatoxin-Initiated Preneoplastic Liver Lesions by Low Dietary Protein," *Nutrition and Cancer* 3 (1982): 200–206.

15. Linda D. Youngman, "The Growth and Development of Aflatoxin B1-Induced Preneoplastic Lesions, Tumors, Metastases, and Spontaneous Tumors as They Are Influenced by Dietary Protein, Level, Type, and Intervention." (Ph.D. dissertation, Cornell University, Ithaca, NY, 1990.)

16. Walter C. Willett et al., "Relation of Meat, Fat, and Fiber Intake to the Risk of Colon Cancer in a Prospective Study Among Women," *New England Journal of Medicine* 323 (1990): 1664–1671.

17. Diana C. Farrow and Scott Davis, "Diet and the Risk of Pancreatic Cancer in Men," *America Journal of Epidemiology* 132 (1990): 423–431.

18. Daniel Fau et al., "Effects of Ingestion of High Protein or Excess Methionine Diets by Rats for Two Years," *Journal of Nutrition* 118 (1988): 128–133.

19. Dean Ornish et al., "Can Lifestyle Changes Reverse Coronary Heart Disease? (The Life-style Heart Trial)," *The Lancet* 336 (1990): 129–133.

Chapter 4: Less Protein, More Health

1. T. Colin Campbell, "A Plant-Enriched Diet and Long-term Health, Particularly in Reference to China." Paper presented at the Second International Symposium on Horticulture and Human Health, Alexandria, Va. (November 4, 1989).
2. Ibid.
3. Fumihiko Horio et al., "Thermogenesis, Low-Protein Diets, and Decreased Development of AFB1-Induced Preneoplastic Foci in Rat Liver," *Nutrition and Cancer* 16 (1991): 31–41.
4. T. Colin Campbell et al., "China: From Diseases of Poverty to Diseases of Affluence. Policy Implications of the Epidemiological Transition." Paper part of NIH Grant 5R01CA33638 (Bethesda, Md.: National Institutes of Health, 1990).
5. Ibid.

Chapter 7: Exercise: Less Pain, More Sane

1. Steven N. Blair et al., "Physical Fitness and All-Cause Mortality: A Prospective Study of Healthy Men and Women," *Journal of the American Medical Association* 262 (1989): 17, 2395–2401.
2. Ibid.
3. American Dietetic Association, "Nutrition and Physical Fitness," *Journal of the American Dietetic Association* 76 (1980): 437.
4. E. H. Christensen and O. Hansen, "Arbeitsfahighkeit und Ehrnahrum," *Scandinavica Archiva Physiologica* 81 (1939): 160–175.
5. J. L. Walberg et al., "Macronutrient Content of a Hypoenergy Diet Affects Nitrogen Retention and Muscle Function in Weight Lifters," *International Journal of Sports Medicine* 9 (1988): 261–266; J. L. Ivy et al., "Muscle Glycogen Storage," *Journal of Applied Physiology* 65 (1988): 2018–2023; M. G. Holl et al., "The Comparative Effect of Meals High in Protein, Sucrose and Starch," *British Journal of Sports Medicine* 22 (1988): 109–111; M. L. Millard-Stafford et al., "The Effect of Glucose Polymer Dietary Supplements with Relation to Swimmers, Cyclists and Runners," *European Journal of Applied Physiology* 58 (1988): 327–333.

Chapter 8: Supplementing Your Low-Protein Diet

1. K. Fred Gey et al., "Plasma Levels of Antioxidant Vitamins in Relation to Ischemic Heart Disease and Cancer," *American Journal of Clinical Nutrition* 45 (1987): 1368–1377.
2. James M. Robertson et al., "Vitamin E Intake and Risk of Cataracts in Humans," *Annals of the New York Academy of Science* 570 (1989): 372–382.
3. Allen Taylor, "Associations Between Nutrition and Cataract," *Nutrition Reviews* 47 (1989): 225–234.

4. Roberta J. Ward et al., "Antioxidant Status in Alcoholic Liver Disease in Man and Experimental Animals," *Biochemical Society Transcripts* 17 (1989): 492.

5. A. Jendryczko and M. Drozdz, "Plasma Retinol, Beta-Carotene and Vitamin E Levels in Relation to the Future Risk of Pre-eclampsia," *Zent. bl. Gynakologica* 111 (1989): 1121–1123.

6. Mohsen Meydani, "Protective Role of Dietary Vitamin E on the Oxidative Stress in Aging," U.S.D.A. Human Nutrition Research Center on Aging at Tufts University. (Paper delivered at 5th Annual Meeting of the American College of Clinical Gerontology, New York, October 1990.)

7. Anthony T. Diplock, "Antioxidant Nutrients and Disease Prevention: An Overview," *American Journal of Clinical Nutrition* 54 (1991): 189S–193S.

8. Cedric F. Garland et al., "Serum-25 hydroxyvitamin D and Colon Cancer: Eight-year Prospective Study," *The Lancet* 2 (1989): 1176–1178.

9. Kenneth W. Kinzler et al., "Identification of a Gene Located at Chromosome 5q21 That Is Mutated in Colorectal Cancers," *Science* 251 (1991): 1366–1370.

10. As reported in *Medical World News*, January 8, 1990.

11. Charles H. Hennekens, "Aspirin in the Primary Prevention of Angina Pectoris in a Randomized Trial of U.S. Physicians," *American Journal of Medicine* 89 (1990): 772–776.

Chapter 9: Extending Your Own Life Span

1. Morris H. Ross et al., "Dietary Habits and the Prediction of Life Span of Rats: A Prospective Test," *American Journal of Clinical Nutrition* 41 (1985): 1332–1344.

2. Clive M. McCay et al., "The Life Span of Rats on a Restricted Diet," *Journal of Nutrition* 18 (1939): 1–25.

3. Byung Pal Yu et al., "Nutritional Influences on Aging of Fischer 344 Rats. 1. Physical, Metabolic and Longevity Characteristics," *Journal of Gerontology* 40 (1985): 657.

4. Richard Hochschild, "Can an Index of Aging Be Constructed for Evaluating Treatments to Retard Aging Rates? A 2,462-Person Study," prepublication (The Hoch Company, 2915 Pebble Drive, Corona del Mar, Ca. 92625).

Chapter 10: The Essential Truth of Anti-Aging

1. Edward L. Schneider and Jack M. Guralnik, "The Aging of America: Impact on Health Care Costs," *Journal of the American Medical Association* 263 (1990): 2335–2355.

2. Joseph D. Beasley and Jerry J. Swift, *The Kellogg Report: The Impact of Nutrition, Environment and Lifestyle on the Health of Americans* (Annandale-on-Hudson, NY 12504: The Institute of Health Policy and Practice, The Bard College Center, 1989), pp. 453–454.

INDEX